# The Plant Based Diet

*This Books Includes: An Essential Guide for Beginners & A Complete Meal Plan with 160 Delicious Recipes*

**SEBI ALAN GUNTRY**

# The Plant Based Diet For Beginners

*A Complete Diet Guide for Beginners for Easy Weight Loss and Burn Fat to Kick-Start a Healthy Lifestyle with a Plant Based Eating in a Few Weeks*

# The Plant Based Diet Meal Plan

*The New Vegetable Diet Cookbook with Vegan, Fat Free Vegan and Low Carbs Recipes to Burn Fat, Stimulate Weight Loss and Energy Reset*

# The Plant Based Diet For Beginners

*A Complete Diet Guide for Beginners for Easy Weight Loss and Burn Fat to Kick-Start a Healthy Lifestyle with a Plant Based Eating in a Few Weeks*

**SEBI ALAN GUNTRY**

# Table of Contents

## CHAPTER 7. THE PLANT BASED SNACKS FOR MORNING AND AFTERNOON...........................146

# Introduction

Selecting the perfect diet plan can be confusing thanks to the variety of diet plans available these days. Irrespective of what diet plan you opt for, almost all nutritionists and dietitians across the globe recommend diet plans that limit processed foods and that are based more on whole and fresh foods. The Plant-Based Diet is based on these universally preferred foods.

This introduction is going to clear away all ambiguities and doubts regarding the whole-food, plant-based diet plan and provide logical explanations to the benefits it offers.

The whole-food plant-based diet plan is more flexible and understanding than other diets, too. It is mostly comprised of plant-based foods, but you can also have some animal-based products.

Now knowing that eating animal products is a huge risk to your health, it definitely stands as a solid reason why you should opt for plant-based foods. Besides improving your overall health, these foods have numerous benefits to your body. First, they are rich in fiber. Therefore, your digestion will be improved. Their high fiber content, however, demands that dieters should slowly change their usual meals because the bodies take time to adapt. This is a worrying statistic, especially bearing in mind that obesity is linked to cardiovascular diseases and diabetes. Adopting a plant-based diet can help in promoting weight loss. The great thing about this is that you will lose weight naturally without having to worry about gaining again in the future. Usually, the fad diets that people rush to rely on have long-term negative effects. Most people complain about gaining more weight after they had initially shed some pounds. Eating plant foods could prevent such effects. A plant-based diet emphasizes the consumption of anything derived from plants - vegetables, cereals, nuts and seeds - minimizing or excluding animal products. While some may think that a plant-based diet is just another term for a vegetarian or even a vegan diet, there is a fundamental difference. Plant-based diets emphasize the consumption of whole and natural foods and avoid processed foods such as tofu, seitan or packaged products, even if they are technically vegan or vegetarian. A diet composed only of plants will be beneficial in maintaining healthy skin. Providing your skin with the nutrients it requires is the best way of keeping it smooth and glowing.

Unfortunately, people lack information about this. As such, they are forced to try different skin products with the hopes of giving their skin a natural glow and clear complexion. Eating right is a solution to almost every disease that we might be suffering from. We have been blinded by the media from realizing that the cure we need is in our food choices.

# *What is a Plant-based diet?*

Though there are variations within a plant-based diet, the major cornerstone of the diet is that plant foods become the central focal point of your diet. This means that you base your meals around food products sourced from plants like vegetables, nuts, seeds, whole grains, fruits, and legumes. Animal products are either cut out completely or are otherwise reduced. How much you reduce your intake of animal products depends upon what you deem best for yourself. However, if you do choose to make animal products such as fish, poultry, meat, dairy, or eggs a part of your diet, they will take a backseat to the plant foods that make up your meals. If this makes you feel nervous, don't worry! This is not a deprivation diet. There are so many appetizing and tasty plant food options out there that you may not even know about! Many of us are so accustomed to meat, animal products and processed foods taking center-stage at meal times that it is hard to imagine what a meal that puts plant foods first would look like. Embarking on a plant-based diet provides you an exciting opportunity to explore new foods and recipes that are not only satisfying and nourishing but are delicious and taste amazing as well.

The following diets all fall under the umbrella of a plant-based diet:

•	Vegan: Diet includes vegetables, seeds, nuts, legumes, grains, and fruit and excludes all animal products (i.e. no animal flesh, dairy, or eggs). There are variations within the vegan diet as well such as the fruitarian diet made up mainly of fruits and sometimes nuts and seeds and the raw vegan diet where food is not cooked.

•	Vegetarian: Diet includes vegetables, fruit, nuts, legumes, grains, and seeds and excludes meat but may include eggs or dairy. The Ovo-lacto vegetarian diet incorporates dairy and eggs while the Ovo-vegetarian diet incorporates eggs and excludes dairy and the lacto vegetarian diet incorporates dairy but excludes eggs.

•	Semi-vegetarianism: Diet is mostly vegetarian but also incorporates some meat and animal products. The macrobiotic diet is a type of semi-vegetarian diet that emphasizes vegetables, beans, whole grains, naturally processed foods, and may include some seafood, meat, or poultry. The pescatarian diet includes plant foods, eggs, dairy, and seafood but no other types of animal flesh. People who subscribe to a semi-vegetarian diet sometimes describe themselves as flexitarians as well.

The plant-based, whole food diet is really all about trying to only consume whole, unrefined plants. Followers of a plant-based diet like to get their food as organically as possible. If the food is refined, it must only be minimally refined. Vegetables, fruits, whole grains, tubers, and legumes are going to be the most important parts of meals and animal products either take a on a small proportion of the meal or are excluded altogether. This includes meat, dairy products, and eggs. Highly refined products like bleached flour, oil, and refined sugar are usually avoided as well.

Some of these plant-based diets are obviously stricter than others. No one diet is right for everyone, so it is important to understand all the options you have within a plant-based diet so that you can choose which lifestyle is most attractive and feels right to you. Maybe you want to cut out all animal products and go vegan, consuming only plant foods and products or maybe you prefer keeping some animal products in your diet while making plant foods your main focus. Remember, you are in control of what you eat and what goes into your body. A plant-based diet will likely have more restrictions and parameters than you are used to, so it is crucial that you pick a diet that is not only healthy, but attainable, realistic to adhere to, and enjoyable for you. The plant-based diet is designed to increase your quality of life so it would be counter-productive to choose a diet that makes you feel deprived or unhappy! It is important to set realistic expectations for yourself so that you are able to follow your new diet and are not tempted to stray from it. That being said, following a plant-based diet can be incredibly easy and simple if you follow the right steps and stay committed to your new healthy choices which will not be hard to do once you start feeling the beneficial effects of this health-focused lifestyle.

There has often been some confusion as to whether the plant based diet is just another word for veganism, or if they are a completely different concept with different rules, so let's go into that. There are many similarities between the two, but also some distinct differences. Are veganism and a plant based diet the same thing? The short answer is no. Like I said before, the particular diet that is chosen and the label it is given depends on the individual, and the reason they have chosen to live this lifestyle. Many vegans choose to be so because they disagree with the slaughter and poor treatment of farm animals, and so they so not consume these foods. They also usually choose not to use leather, or wear fur or any other animal products. Vegans do not eat any sort of meat, or product containing traces of meat. This includes any broths, or ingredients such as gelatin. Vegans also do not eat any food products that contain ANY ingredient from an animal, including milk or honey. They do not eat any cheese, or yogurt, or margarine or butter, etc. Some slightly more hidden ingredients that contain animal product are whey and casein. These are all avoided. Vegans get most of their food from plant sources, but they are not strictly whole food plant based. They may not be as health conscious, and so many may choose to eat packaged and processed foods yet stay away from those made of animal. This technically still falls within the parameter of their diet.

Plant based folks eat a primarily plant derived diet-as close to nature as possible. But this does not mean that they are vegan, or even vegetarian. They may simply choose to eat mostly fruits, vegetables, nuts and legumes, etc. However, they may still choose to eat meat, and carefully choose meats that are antibiotics free, grass fed, and lived a free-range life. Many plant based dieters believe that meat is still an integral part of a healthy diet, and so they just choose the best quality possible.

Whole food, plant based diets usually take the qualities of both diets, and even go a step further. Keeping foods whole refers to leaving them in their most natural state. So, vegetables and fruit are eaten as they are-fresh, frozen or dried without preservatives or added flavor. Nuts are natural, without salt or sugar; grains are not refined or enriched or bleached. Most foods are prepared at home, or in a restaurant where they chefs share the same standards, as to not degrade any of the ingredients or take away any of their nutritional value. Many processed foods use what is known as plant fragments, rather than whole plants. They are reduced or extracted or otherwise processed in some way. Whatever the specifics of the diet someone chooses, if they tell you that they are vegan or plant based, you should assume that they do not consume any animal products at all, unless they mention it otherwise. This can help you to avoid accidentally serving them something that they will not be willing or able to eat. And feel free to ask someone about their diet, if you are curious. But make sure that they are willing to talk about it, and also that you listen with an open mind-not looking to judge or challenge their decision to adopt that particular diet.

Now, I would like to clarify the way in which I am using the word diet here. I know that many diets are short term and involve cutting calories and foods in order to lose unwanted weight. This is a bit of a touchy thing, because there are many diets out there which can put extreme pressure on the body and will cause weight loss through force or a particular calculation or schedule of eating. This is not what I am referring to in this book. What I will be proposing is that you, the reader, adopt a new addition to your lifestyle that will benefit you, and that you can stick with permanently. This may sound a bit intimidating, to adopt new eating rules for life. However, it is my hope that with my help, you will be able to do this painlessly, and really see benefits from it. You may lose weight; you may have clearer skin and eyes, healthier hair, and even have more abundant energy. And you will help to determine just which benefits you will be rewarded with, by deciding how far you want to go.

Benefits of Plant Based Diet

A plant-based diet has significant benefits of improving health and being eco-friendlier. Some of the benefits are as follows:

Weight Loss and Overall Improved Health

Obesity is one of the significant health issues faced by the majority of people these days, ranging from children to old. Proper diet changes can lead to radical weight loss, which would be promising and long-lasting. Various studies report that effective weight loss can be achieved with the help of plant-based diet plans.

The plant-based diet plan is ideal for weight loss, as it is rich in proteins and fiber, limits processed foods, and forbids refined grains, soda, candy, fast food, and added sugars. According to a few research reports, plant-based diet followers lose weight more quickly as compared to non-plant-based diet followers. Weight loss from a plant-based diet plan is quite long-lasting with improved health.

Beneficial in Various Health Issues

In addition to weight loss, a plant-based diet helps to

reduce the menaces of numerous chronic health conditions.

Cardiac Conditions

The foremost benefit of a plant-based diet plan is that it keeps the cardiac health sound, depending upon the quality and types of the food in your diet plan. Research studies report that the risk of cardiac diseases was lower in those people who follow a plant-based diet that was rich in veggies, whole grains, nuts, fruits, and legumes, as compared to followers of other diets. Plant-based diet plans, including refined grains, sugary drinks, and fruit juices, are very unhealthy and contribute to severe cardiac complications. So, it is essential to follow a healthy plant-based diet plan.

Cancer

Research studies report that a plant-based diet plan can avoid various forms of cancer. The risks of gastrointestinal and colorectal cancers are reported to be significantly reduced amongst plant-based diet followers.

Cognitive Decline

According to some studies, Alzheimer's disease and

cognitive decline can be prevented in adults with the help of diet plans high in veggie and fruit content due to a large number of antioxidants and other compounds. Consumption of more fruits and vegetables leads to a 20 percent lower risk of having dementia or cognitive impairment.

## Diabetes

In order to reduce the risk of contracting diabetes, one should consider following a plant-based diet plan. Followers of the plant-based diet plan mitigate the risk of having diabetes by 34 percent when compared to followers of other diets. Fifty percent reduction of type 2 diabetes was observed amongst the followers of Lacto-Ovo vegetarian and vegan diet plans. Blood sugar level control is highly improved in the diabetic followers of plant-based diet plans.

## Eco-friendlier Diet

In addition to benefits in health, a plant-based diet plan has proved to be advantageous for the ecosystem, as they have little effect on the environment as compared to other diet plan followers. A plant-based diet helps in the minimization of global warming, as it results in a 50-

70 percent reduction in greenhouse gas emissions, land usage, and lower water usage. A plant-based diet also helps in boosting the economy due to lower dependency on unsustainable practices like factory farming and reduction in animal-based food.

# *Plant-Based Diet for Weight Loss*

It is a natural fact that only through watching what we eat, will we have the most impact on our weight. This is where the plant-based diet really shines and lets you enjoy automatic, effortless fat burning without all the usual calorie constraints of other diets.

Weight loss is an almost certain result you will enjoy once you start the plant-based diet, but this is not the only benefit that you will enjoy. Think of all those activities you have always wanted to pursue but shelved because you simply had no energy left after your usual day's work.

Well, time to dust off those hobbies and the things you enjoy doing, because on the plant-based, you will have more energy for your daily work and play! The accompanying mental clarity and sharpness of thought are also positive effects which you will have as a direct result of the diet. A better health report card, by way of optimized cholesterol readings, normalized blood sugar and a corresponding lowered risk of cardiovascular diseases are also just some of the beneficial health effects experienced by most on the diet.

Something that many learn is that a diet is almost only as good as the number of recipes it has in its repertoire. The benefits of a particular diet may be numerous, but if you are forced to have the same stuff every breakfast, lunch and dinner, even the most avid supporter of the lot would probably have problems sustaining the diet. This is where I am most happy to say that the plant-based diet has quite some leeway for the concoction of various different recipes, and it is the purpose of this book to bring you some of the more delicious and easy-to-prepare meals for your gastronomic pleasure!

For the beginners as well as the adepts, the recipes contained within are created specifically to be appealing to your palate while not requiring you to literally spend the whole day in the kitchen! Concise and to the point, the recipes break down meal prep. requirements in a simple step by step format, easy for anyone to understand. An additional 21-day meal plan is also structured to serve both as guidance as well as inspiration for the new and old adherents to the diet.

**Don't forget to exercise**

It has always been said that dieting is an effective way to lose weight. However, to keep the weight off, exercise is required. Many studies have shown that exercising while dieting is actually the best way to lose weight. Firstly, the diet becomes more effective and you lose weight faster if you exercise. But it also gets you in the habit of continuing your exercise when your diet is complete.

The exercise expected is not something that is not achievable either. Even with just forty-five minutes of exercise each day, can increase your weight loss by over ten percent! Anything that can get your heartbeat pulsing higher and faster than normal is considered exercise.

Often times, dieting will make you lose weight in many parts that you don't want to lose weight in, such as curvaceous or softening lines. Studies have shown that combined with exercise, dieting can help reduce your body mass index, waist circumference, and percentage of body fat.

Another concern is that with dieting, often times you appear lighter because your muscle and bone density is reduced. That is not a healthy lifestyle in the long term. Exercising will stimulate the growth of your muscles and have your body burn the fat instead of your metabolic tissues.

It is also important to understand that the idea behind dieting is that most people want to look skinnier and overall better. However, lean is what will make you look perfect! Being lean will highlight your figure and keep your body healthy and toned. Skinny means that you have lost a lot of muscle density and water retention. In the long run, it can affect your calcium, iron, and zinc levels in your body.

## Kick-starting your weight-loss journey

To get things done the right way and to ensure your body benefits from this diet, it is essential to consider the following things prior to starting this regimen.

## Well Organized Meal plan

Please note that the main purpose of this book and diet plan is to help you lose weight and help in maintaining a healthy lifestyle. Because of this, you have to follow a strict plan to achieve your goals. This book provides a 21-day plant-based plan to kick-start your wellness journey. Please remember that this meal plan will require some commitment, and it is not how your diet will always be structured after the 21-day plan. After 21 days, once your body has adjusted, you will be able to make a consistent meal plan schedule where fasting is not required.

## Understand Your Body

Getting your blood tested for the existence of any underlying condition is important to ensure that you start the regimen without worrying about it affecting your health negatively. Though, it doesn't harm your body, but in case you are suffering from a serious condition, it is best that you don't go on any sort of weight loss diet.

It is important to get your blood tested for lipid panel, liver and kidney function, inflammatory markers, thyroid panel and blood count.

## Get enough sleep and relax efficiently

It is important that you understand that you must take this diet easy and relax while practicing it. Your goal must not be to quickly cut down your carb intake, so you can lose an enormous amount of your body weight as soon as possible. Rather, you should reduce it slowly and gradually. Don't worry; you will still benefit a lot from this plan. Going easy on yourself helps you experience less side effects and enables your body to adjust comfortably to the completely new diet plan.

**Get Professional Support**

It is wise to get the assistance of a professional healthcare practitioner, dietician, or nutritionist who can help you out in preparing good meal plans for you. In this case, this e-book will do this job for you by providing you with more meal plans and guidance in the next series. Nonetheless, it is a good idea to consult a professional at least once before commencing the diet just to make sure that you know your body is ready for it. You will also find it easier to prepare good meal plans that are customized just for you.

In case, you suffer from heart diseases or other conditions such as epilepsy, HBP, diabetes (TYPE 2), Alzheimer's or any other medical condition, then it is absolutely essential for you to get a professional's help before and during the plan.

**Create time**

This is one of the most crucial factors to consider before implementing the low-carb diet. You must not start it when you are going through an extremely hectic schedule and have no time to spare for yourself. This is because this diet demands you to prepare special meals and get used to different foods that you aren't accustomed to eating regularly. These changes will stress you out, so you need to have enough time to devote to this new routine, at least for about two weeks.

Therefore, you must start the plant-based diet when you are emotionally, psychologically, and physically relaxed and free.

**Be careful with other people's opinions**

If you are to achieve optimal this goal, you will definitely need to understand that you cannot just eat anything even when in social places otherwise you will end up jeopardizing your entire regime since it takes time for any carbs you take to be completely out of your body. As such, you should be psychologically prepared to take different foods that might attract some attention and well-meaning but often misleading comments about the diet. Being prepared will ensure you don't give up.

**Recipes**

By now, you should have enough info to start your plant-based diet plan. In the subsequent chapters, we will discuss what your eating schedule should look like throughout your first four weeks of starting. This will ensure you start the diet correctly and be well on your way to losing excess weight quickly and eating healthy. This book comes with more than 50 pre-designed ketogenic diet recipes to get you started! There's a recipes section after the weekly diet plans, so keep reading.

# *The Plant Based Breakfast*

**Hot Pink Smoothie**

Preparation time: 5 minutes

Cooking time: 0 minute

Servings: 1

Ingredients:

1 clementine, peeled, segmented

1/2 frozen banana

1 small beet, peeled, chopped

1/8 teaspoon sea salt

1/2 cup raspberries

1 tablespoon chia seeds

1/4 teaspoon vanilla extract, unsweetened

2 tablespoons almond butter

1 cup almond milk, unsweetened

Method:

Place all the ingredients in the order in a food processor or blender and then pulse for 2 to 3 minutes at high speed until smooth.

Pour the smoothie into a glass and then serve.

Nutrition Value:

Calories: 278 Cal

Fat: 5.6 g

Carbs: 37.2 g

Protein: 6.2 g

Fiber: 13.2 g


**Maca Caramel Frap**

Preparation time: 5 minutes

Cooking time: 0 minute

Servings: 4

Ingredients:

1/2 of frozen banana, sliced

1/4 cup cashews, soaked for 4 hours

2 Medjool dates, pitted

1 teaspoon maca powder

1/8 teaspoon sea salt

1/2 teaspoon vanilla extract, unsweetened

1/4 cup almond milk, unsweetened

1/4 cup cold coffee, brewed

Method:

Place all the ingredients in the order in a food processor or blender and then pulse for 2 to 3 minutes at high speed until smooth.

Pour the smoothie into a glass and then serve.

Nutrition Value:

Calories: 450 Cal

Fat: 170 g

Carbs: 64 g

Protein: 7 g

Fiber: 0 g

## Peanut Butter Vanilla Green Shake

Preparation time: 5 minutes

Cooking time: 0 minute

Servings: 1

Ingredients:

1 teaspoon flax seeds

1 frozen banana

1 cup baby spinach

1/8 teaspoon sea salt

1/2 teaspoon ground cinnamon

1/4 teaspoon vanilla extract, unsweetened

2 tablespoons peanut butter, unsweetened

1/4 cup ice

1 cup coconut milk, unsweetened

Method:

Place all the ingredients in the order in a food processor or blender and then pulse for 2 to 3 minutes at high speed until smooth.

Pour the smoothie into a glass and then serve.

Nutrition Value:

Calories: 298 Cal

Fat: 11 g

Carbs: 32 g

Protein: 24 g

Fiber: 8 g

**Green Colada**

Preparation time: 5 minutes

Cooking time: 0 minute

Servings: 1

Ingredients:

1/2 cup frozen pineapple chunks

1/2 banana

1/2 teaspoon spirulina powder

1/4 teaspoon vanilla extract, unsweetened

1 cup of coconut milk

Method:

Place all the ingredients in the order in a food processor or blender and then pulse for 2 to 3 minutes at high speed until smooth.

Pour the smoothie into a glass and then serve.

Nutrition Value:

Calories: 127 Cal

Fat: 3 g

Carbs: 25 g

Protein: 3 g

Fiber: 4 g

## Chocolate Oat Smoothie

Preparation time: 5 minutes

Cooking time: 0 minute

Servings: 1

Ingredients:

¼ cup rolled oats

1 ½ tablespoon cocoa powder, unsweetened

1 teaspoon flax seeds

1 large frozen banana

1/8 teaspoon sea salt

1/8 teaspoon cinnamon

¼ teaspoon vanilla extract, unsweetened

2 tablespoons almond butter

1 cup coconut milk, unsweetened

Method:

Place all the ingredients in the order in a food processor or blender and then pulse for 2 to 3 minutes at high speed until smooth.

Pour the smoothie into a glass and then serve.

Nutrition Value:

Calories: 262 Cal

Fat: 7.3 g

Carbs: 50.4 g

Protein: 8.1 g

Fiber: 9.6 g

**Peach Crumble Shake**

Preparation time: 5 minutes

Cooking time: 0 minute

Servings: 1

Ingredients:

1 tablespoon chia seeds

¼ cup rolled oats

2 peaches, pitted, sliced

¾ teaspoon ground cinnamon

1 Medjool date, pitted

½ teaspoon vanilla extract, unsweetened

2 tablespoons lemon juice

½ cup of water

1 tablespoon coconut butter

1 cup coconut milk, unsweetened

Method:

Place all the ingredients in the order in a food processor or blender and then pulse for 2 to 3 minutes at high speed until smooth.

Pour the smoothie into a glass and then serve.

Nutrition Value:

Calories: 270 Cal

Fat: 4 g

Carbs: 28 g

Protein: 25 g

Fiber: 3 g

## Wild Ginger Green Smoothie

Preparation time: 5 minutes

Cooking time: 0 minute

Servings: 1

Ingredients:

1/2 cup pineapple chunks, frozen

1/2 cup chopped kale

1/2 frozen banana

1 tablespoon lime juice

2 inches ginger, peeled, chopped

1/2 cup coconut milk, unsweetened

1/2 cup coconut water

Method:

Place all the ingredients in the order in a food processor or blender and then pulse for 2 to 3 minutes at high speed until smooth.

Pour the smoothie into a glass and then serve.

Nutrition Value:

Calories: 331 Cal

Fat: 14 g

Carbs: 40 g

Protein: 16 g

Fiber: 9 g


**Berry Beet Velvet Smoothie**

Preparation time: 5 minutes

Cooking time: 0 minute

Servings: 1

Ingredients:

1/2 of frozen banana

1 cup mixed red berries

1 Medjool date, pitted

1 small beet, peeled, chopped

1 tablespoon cacao powder

1 teaspoon chia seeds

1/4 teaspoon vanilla extract, unsweetened

1/2 teaspoon lemon juice

2 teaspoons coconut butter

1 cup coconut milk, unsweetened

Method:

Place all the ingredients in the order in a food processor or blender and then pulse for 2 to 3 minutes at high speed until smooth.

Pour the smoothie into a glass and then serve.

Nutrition Value:

Calories: 234 Cal

Fat: 5 g

Carbs: 42 g

Protein: 11 g

Fiber: 7 g

**Spiced Strawberry Smoothie**

Preparation time: 5 minutes

Cooking time: 0 minute

Servings: 1

Ingredients:

1 tablespoon goji berries, soaked

1 cup strawberries

1/8 teaspoon sea salt

1 frozen banana

1 Medjool date, pitted

1 scoop vanilla-flavored whey protein

2 tablespoons lemon juice

¼ teaspoon ground ginger

½ teaspoon ground cinnamon

1 tablespoon almond butter

1 cup almond milk, unsweetened

Method:

Place all the ingredients in the order in a food processor or blender and then pulse for 2 to 3 minutes at high speed until smooth.

Pour the smoothie into a glass and then serve.

Nutrition Value:

Calories: 182 Cal

Fat: 1.3 g

Carbs: 34 g

Protein: 6.4 g

Fiber: 0.7 g


**Banana Bread Shake With Walnut Milk**

Preparation time: 5 minutes

Cooking time: 0 minute

Servings: 2

Ingredients:

2 cups sliced frozen bananas

3 cups walnut milk

1/8 teaspoon grated nutmeg

1 tablespoon maple syrup

1 teaspoon ground cinnamon

1/2 teaspoon vanilla extract, unsweetened

2 tablespoons cacao nibs

Method:

Place all the ingredients in the order in a food processor or blender and then pulse for 2 to 3 minutes at high speed until smooth.

Pour the smoothie into two glasses and then serve.

Nutrition Value:

Calories: 339.8 Cal

Fat: 19 g

Carbs: 39 g

Protein: 4.3 g

Fiber: 1 g

## Double Chocolate Hazelnut Espresso Shake

Preparation time: 5 minutes

Cooking time: 0 minute

Servings: 1

Ingredients:

1 frozen banana, sliced

1/4 cup roasted hazelnuts

4 Medjool dates, pitted, soaked

2 tablespoons cacao nibs, unsweetened

1 1/2 tablespoons cacao powder, unsweetened

1/8 teaspoon sea salt

1 teaspoon vanilla extract, unsweetened

1 cup almond milk, unsweetened

1/2 cup ice

4 ounces espresso, chilled

Method:

Place all the ingredients in the order in a food processor or blender and then pulse for 2 to 3 minutes at high speed until smooth.

Pour the smoothie into a glass and then serve.

Nutrition Value:

Calories: 210 Cal

Fat: 5 g

Carbs: 27 g

Protein: 16.8 g

Fiber: 0.2 g

## Strawberry, Banana and Coconut Shake

Preparation time: 5 minutes

Cooking time: 0 minute

Servings: 1

Ingredients:

1 tablespoon coconut flakes

1 1/2 cups frozen banana slices

8 strawberries, sliced

1/2 cup coconut milk, unsweetened

1/4 cup strawberries for topping

Method:

Place all the ingredients in the order in a food processor or blender, except for topping and then pulse for 2 to 3 minutes at high speed until smooth.

Pour the smoothie into a glass and then serve.

Nutrition Value:

Calories: 335 Cal

Fat: 5 g

Carbs: 75 g

Protein: 4 g

Fiber: 9 g

## Tropical Vibes Green Smoothie

Preparation time: 5 minutes

Cooking time: 0 minute

Servings: 1

Ingredients:

2 stalks of kale, ripped

1 frozen banana

1 mango, peeled, pitted, chopped

1/8 teaspoon sea salt

¼ cup of coconut yogurt

½ teaspoon vanilla extract, unsweetened

1 tablespoon ginger juice

½ cup of orange juice

½ cup of coconut water

Method:

Place all the ingredients in the order in a food processor or blender and then pulse for 2 to 3 minutes at high speed until smooth.

Pour the smoothie into a glass and then serve.

Nutrition Value:

Calories: 197.5 Cal

Fat: 1.3 g

Carbs: 30 g

Protein: 16.3 g

Fiber: 4.8 g

## Peanut Butter and Mocha Smoothie

Preparation time: 5 minutes

Cooking time: 0 minute

Servings: 1

Ingredients:

1 frozen banana, chopped

1 scoop of chocolate protein powder

2 tablespoons rolled oats

1/8 teaspoon sea salt

¼ teaspoon vanilla extract, unsweetened

1 teaspoon cocoa powder, unsweetened

2 tablespoons peanut butter

1 shot of espresso

½ cup almond milk, unsweetened

Method:

Place all the ingredients in the order in a food processor or blender and then pulse for 2 to 3 minutes at high speed until smooth.

Pour the smoothie into a glass and then serve.

Nutrition Value:

Calories: 380 Cal

Fat: 14 g

Carbs: 29 g

Protein: 38 g

Fiber: 4 g

**Tahini Shake with Cinnamon and Lime**

Preparation time: 5 minutes

Cooking time: 0 minute

Servings: 1

Ingredients:

1 frozen banana

2 tablespoons tahini

1/8 teaspoon sea salt

¾ teaspoon ground cinnamon

¼ teaspoon vanilla extract, unsweetened

2 teaspoons lime juice

1 cup almond milk, unsweetened

Method:

Place all the ingredients in the order in a food processor or blender and then pulse for 2 to 3 minutes at high speed until smooth.

Pour the smoothie into a glass and then serve.

Nutrition Value:

Calories: 225 Cal

Fat: 15 g

Carbs: 22 g

Protein: 6 g

Fiber: 8 g


**Fig Oatmeal Bake**

Preparation time: 5 minutes

Cooking time: 15 minutes

Servings: 4

Ingredients:

2 fresh figs, sliced

5 dried figs, chopped

4 tablespoons chopped walnuts

1 ½ cups oats

1 teaspoon cinnamon

2 tablespoons agave syrup

1 teaspoon baking powder

2 tablespoons unsalted butter, melted

3 tablespoons flaxseed egg

¾ cup of coconut milk

Directions:

Switch on the oven, then set it to 350 degrees F and let it preheat.

Meanwhile, take a bowl, place all the ingredients in it, except for fresh figs and stir until combined.

Take an 8-inch square pan, line it with parchment sheet, spoon in the prepared mixture, top with fig slices, and bake for 30 minutes until cooked and set.

Serve straight away

Nutrition:

Calories: 372.8 Cal

Fat: 9.2 g

Carbs: 65.6 g

Protein: 11.6 g

Fiber: 11.1 g

**Vegan Breakfast Sandwich**

Preparation time: 15 minutes

Cooking time: 8 minutes

Servings: 3

Ingredients:

1 cup of spinach

6 slices of pickle

14 oz tofu, extra-firm, pressed

2 medium tomatoes, sliced

1/2 teaspoon garlic powder

¼ teaspoon ground black pepper

1/2 teaspoon black salt

1 teaspoon turmeric

1 tablespoon coconut oil

2 tablespoons vegan mayo

3 slices of vegan cheese

6 slices of gluten-free bread, toasted

Directions:

Cut tofu into six slices, and then season its one side with garlic, black pepper, salt, and turmeric.

Take a skillet pan, place it over medium heat, add oil and when hot, add seasoned tofu slices in it, season side down, and Cooking Time: for 3 minutes until crispy and light brown.

Then flip the tofu slices and continue cooking for 3 minutes until browned and crispy.

When done, transfer tofu slices on a baking sheet, in the form of a set of two slices side by side, then top each set with a cheese slice and broil for 3 minutes until cheese has melted.

Spread mayonnaise on both sides of slices, top with two slices of tofu, cheese on the side, top with spinach, tomatoes, pickles, and then close the sandwich.

Cut the sandwich into half and then serve.

Nutrition:

Calories: 364 Cal

Fat: 12 g

Carbs: 51 g

Protein: 16 g

Fiber: 3 g

**Vegan Fried Egg**

Preparation time: 5 minutes

Cooking time: 8 minutes

Servings: 4

Ingredients:

1 block of firm tofu, firm, pressed, drained

½ teaspoon ground black pepper

½ teaspoon salt

1 tablespoon vegan butter

1 cup vegan toast dipping sauce

Directions:

Cut tofu into four slices, and then shape them into a rough circle by using a cookie cutter.

Take a frying pan, place it over medium heat, add butter and when it melts, add prepared tofu slices in a single layer and Cooking Time: for 3 minutes per side until light brown.

Transfer tofu to serving dishes, make a small hole in the middle of tofu by using a small cookie cutter and fill the hole with dipping sauce.

Garnish eggs with black pepper and sauce and then serve.

Nutrition:

Calories: 86 Cal

Fat: 9 g

Carbs: 0.5 g

Protein: 2 g

Fiber: 0 g

## Sweet Crepes

Preparation time: 5 minutes

Cooking time: 8 minutes

Servings: 5

Ingredients:

1 cup of water

1 banana

1/2 cup oat flour

1/2 cup brown rice flour

1 teaspoon baking powder

1 tablespoon coconut sugar

1/8 teaspoon salt

Directions:

Take a blender, place all the ingredients in it except for sugar and salt and pulse for 1 minute until smooth.

Take a skillet pan, place it over medium-high heat, grease it with oil and when hot, pour in ¼ cup of batter, spread it as thin as possible, and Cooking Time: for 2 to 3 minutes per side until golden brown.

Cooking Time: remaining crepes in the same manner, then sprinkle with sugar and salt and serve.

Nutrition:

Calories: 160.1 Cal

Fat: 4.3 g

Carbs: 22 g

Protein: 8.3 g

Fiber: 0.6 g

**Spinach Artichoke Quiche**

Preparation time: 10 minutes

Cooking time: 55 minutes

Servings: 4

Ingredients:

14 oz tofu, soft

14 oz of artichokes, chopped

2 cups spinach

½ of a large onion, peeled, chopped

1 lemon, juiced

1 teaspoon minced garlic

¼ teaspoon salt

¼ teaspoon ground black pepper

1 teaspoon dried basil

½ teaspoon turmeric

1 tablespoon coconut oil

1 teaspoon Dijon mustard

½ cup nutritional yeast

2 large tortillas, cut into half

Directions:

Switch on the oven, then set it to 350 degrees F and let it preheat.

Take a pie plate, grease it with oil, place tortilla to cover the bottom and sides of the plate and bake for 10 to 15 minutes until baked.

Meanwhile, take a large pan, place it over medium heat, add oil and when hot, add onion and Cooking Time: for 5 minutes.

Then add garlic, Cooking Time: for 1 minute until fragrant, stir in spinach and Cooking Time: for 4 minutes until the spinach has wilted, set aside when done.

Place tofu in a food processor, add all the spices, yeast, and lemon juice and pulse for 2 minutes until smooth.

Then add cooked onion mixture and artichokes, blend for 15 to 25 times until combined, and then pour the mixture over crust in the pie plate.

Bake quiche for 45 minutes until done, then cut it into wedges and serve.

Nutrition:

Calories: 100.3 Cal

Fat: 4.7 g

Carbs: 5 g

Protein: 9.3 g

Fiber: 0.7 g

**Tofu Scramble**

Preparation time: 5 minutes

Cooking time: 18 minutes

Servings: 4

Ingredients:

For The Spice Mix:

1 teaspoon black salt

1/4 teaspoon garlic powder

1 teaspoon red chili powder

1 teaspoon ground cumin

3/4 teaspoons turmeric

2 tablespoons nutritional yeast

For The Tofu Scramble:

2 cups cooked black beans

16 ounces tofu, firm, pressed, drained

1 chopped red pepper

1 1/2 cups sliced button mushrooms

1/2 of white onion, chopped

1 teaspoon minced garlic

1 tablespoon olive oil

Directions:

Take a skillet pan, place it over medium-high heat, add oil and when hot, add onion, pepper, mushrooms, and garlic and Cooking Time: for 8 minutes until golden.

Meanwhile, prepare the spice mix and for this, place all its ingredients in a bowl and stir until combined.

When vegetables have cooked, add tofu in it, crumble it, then add black beans, sprinkle with prepared spice mix, stir and Cooking Time: for 8 minutes until hot.

Serve straight away

Nutrition:

Calories: 175 Cal

Fat: 9 g

Carbs: 10 g

Protein: 14 g

Fiber: 3 g

**Pumpkin Muffins**

Preparation time: 15 minutes

Cooking time: 30 minutes

Servings: 9

Ingredients:

2 Tablespoon mashed ripe banana

1.5 flax eggs

1 teaspoon vanilla extract, unsweetened

1/4 cup maple syrup

1/4 cup olive oil

2/3 cup coconut sugar

3/4 cup pumpkin puree

1 1/4 teaspoon pumpkin pie spice

1/4 teaspoon sea salt

1/2 teaspoon ground cinnamon

2 teaspoon baking soda

1/2 cup water

1/2 cup almond meal

1 cup gluten-free flour blend

3/4 cup rolled oats

For the Crumble:

2 Tablespoon chopped pecans

3 1/2 Tablespoon gluten-free flour blend

3 Tablespoon coconut sugar

1/8 teaspoon cinnamon

1/8 teaspoon pumpkin pie spice

1 1/4 Tablespoon coconut oil

Directions:

Switch on the oven, then set it to 350 degrees F and let it preheat.

Meanwhile, prepare the muffin batter and for this, place the first seven ingredients in a bowl and whisk until combined.

Then whisk in the next five ingredients until mixed and gradually beat in remaining ingredients until incorporated and smooth batter comes together.

Prepare crumble, and for this, place all of its ingredients in a bowl and stir until combined.

Distribute the batter evenly between ten muffin tins lined with muffin liners, top with prepared crumble, and then bake for 30 minutes until muffins are set and the tops are golden brown.

When done, let muffin cool for 5 minutes, then take them out to cool completely and serve.

Nutrition:

Calories: 329 Cal

Fat: 12.7 g

Carbs: 52.6 g

Protein: 4.6 g

Fiber: 5 g

**Tomato and Asparagus Quiche**

Preparation time: 40 minutes

Cooking time: 35 minutes

Servings: 12

Ingredients:

For the Dough:

2 cups whole wheat flour

1/2 teaspoon salt

3/4 cup vegan margarine

1/3 cup water

For the Filling:

14 oz silken tofu

6 cherry tomatoes, halved

2 green onions, cut into rings

10 sun-dried tomatoes, in oil, chopped

7 oz green asparagus, diced

1 1/2 tablespoons herbs de Provence

1 tablespoon cornstarch

1 teaspoon turmeric

3 tablespoons olive oil

Directions:

Switch on the oven, then set it to 350 degrees F and let it preheat.

Pre the dough and for this, take a bowl, place all the ingredients for it, beat until incorporated, then knead for 5 minutes until smooth and refrigerate the dough for 30 minutes.

Meanwhile, take a skillet pan, place it over medium heat, add 1 tablespoon oil and when hot, add green onion and Cooking Time: for 2 minutes, set aside until required.

Place a pot half full wit salty water over medium heat, bring it to boil, then add asparagus and boil for 3 minutes until tender, drain and set aside until required.

Take a medium bowl, add tofu along with herbs de Provence, starch, turmeric, and oil, whisk until smooth and then fold in tomatoes, green onion, and asparagus until mixed.

Divide the prepared dough into twelve sections, take a muffin tray, line it twelve cups with baking cups, and then press a dough ball at the bottom of each cup and all the way up.

Fill the cups with prepared tofu mixture, top with tomatoes, and bake for 35 minutes until cooked.

Serve straight away.

Nutrition:

Calories: 206 Cal

Fat: 14 g

Carbs: 16 g

Protein: 4 g

Fiber: 2 g

**Simple Vegan Breakfast Hash**

Preparation time: 10 minutes

Cooking time: 25 minutes

Servings: 4

Ingredients:

For The Potatoes:

1 large sweet potato, peeled, diced

3 medium potatoes, peeled, diced

1 tablespoon onion powder

2 teaspoons sea salt

1 tablespoon garlic powder

1 teaspoon ground black pepper

1 teaspoon dried thyme

1/4 cup olive oil

For The Skillet Mixture:

1 medium onion, peeled, diced

5 cloves of garlic, peeled, minced

¼ teaspoon of sea salt

¼ teaspoon ground black pepper

1 teaspoon olive oil

Directions:

Switch on the oven, then set it to 450 degrees F and let it preheat.

Meanwhile, take a casserole dish, add all the ingredients for the potatoes, toss until coated, and then Cooking Time: for 20 minutes until crispy, stirring halfway.

Meanwhile, take a skillet pan, place it over medium heat, add oil and when hot, add onion and garlic, season with salt and black pepper and Cooking Time: for 5 minutes until browned.

When potatoes have roasted, add garlic and cooked onion mixture, stir until combined, and serve.

Nutrition:

Calories: 212 Cal

Fat: 10 g

Carbs: 28 g

Protein: 3 g

Fiber: 4 g

**Chickpeas On Toast**

Preparation time: 5 minutes

Cooking time: 15 minutes

Servings: 6

Ingredients:

14-oz cooked chickpeas

1 cup baby spinach

1/2 cup chopped white onion

1 cup crushed tomatoes

½ teaspoon minced garlic

¼ teaspoon ground black pepper

1/2 teaspoon brown sugar

1 teaspoon smoked paprika powder

1/3 teaspoon sea salt

1 tablespoon olive oil

6 slices of gluten-free bread, toasted

Directions:

Take a frying pan, place it over medium heat, add oil and when hot, add onion and Cooking Time: for 2 minutes.

Then stir in garlic, Cooking Time: for 30 seconds until fragrant, stir in paprika and continue cooking for 10 seconds.

Add tomatoes, stir, bring the mixture to simmer, season with black pepper, sugar, and salt and then stir in chickpeas.

Sir, in spinach, Cooking Time: for 2 minutes until leaves have wilted, then remove the pan from heat and taste to adjust seasoning.

Serve cooked chickpeas on toasted bread.

Nutrition:

Calories: 305 Cal

Fat: 7.6 g

Carbs: 45 g

Protein: 13 g

Fiber: 8 g

**Blueberry Muffins**

Preparation time: 5 minutes

Cooking time: 15 minutes

Servings: 12

Ingredients:

2 cups fresh blueberries

2 cups all-purpose flour

2½ teaspoons baking powder

½ teaspoon salt

¼ teaspoon baking soda

½ cup and 2tablespoon. sugar

zest of 1 lemon

1 teaspoon apple cider vinegar

¼ cup and 2 tablespoons. canola oil

1 cup of soy milk

1 teaspoon vanilla extract, unsweetened

Directions:

Switch on the oven, then set it to 450 degrees F and let it preheat.

Meanwhile, take a small bowl, add vinegar and milk, whisk until combined, and let it stand to curdle.

Take a large bowl, add flour, salt, baking powder, and soda, and stir until mixed.

Whisk in sugar, lemon zest, oil, and vanilla into soy milk mixture, then gradually whisk in flour mixture until incorporated and fold in berries until combined.

Take a twelve cups muffin tray, grease them with oil, distribute the prepared batter in them and bake for 25 minutes until done and the tops are browned.

Let muffins cool for 5 minutes, then cool them completely and serve.

Nutrition:

Calories: 160 Cal

Fat: 5 g

Carbs: 25 g

Protein: 2 g

Fiber: 2 g

## Ultimate Breakfast Sandwich

Preparation time: 40 minutes

Cooking time: 10 minutes

Servings: 4

Ingredients:

For the Tofu:

12 ounces tofu, extra-firm, pressed, drain

1/2 teaspoon garlic powder

1 teaspoon liquid smoke

2 tablespoons nutritional yeast

1 teaspoon Sriracha sauce

2 tablespoons soy sauce

2 tablespoons olive oil

2 tablespoons water

For the Vegan Breakfast Sandwich:

1 large tomato, sliced

4 English muffins, halved, toasted

1 avocado, mashed

Directions:

Prepare tofu, and for this, cut tofu into four slices and set aside.

Stir together remaining ingredients of tofu, pour the mixture into a bag, then add tofu pieces, toss until coated and marinate for 30 minutes.

Take a skillet pan, place it over medium-high heat, add tofu slices along with the marinade and Cooking Time: for 5 minutes per side.

Prepare sandwich and for this, spread mashed avocado on the inner of the muffin, top with a slice of tofu, layer with a tomato slice and then serve.

Nutrition:

Calories: 277 Cal

Fat: 9.1 g

Carbs: 33.1 g

Protein: 16.1 g

Fiber: 3.6 g

**Waffles with Fruits**

Preparation time: 10 minutes

Cooking time: 20 minutes

Servings: 4

Ingredients:

1 1/4 cup all-purpose flour

2 teaspoon baking powder

3 tablespoon sugar

1/4 teaspoon salt

2 teaspoon vanilla extract, unsweetened

2 tablespoon coconut oil

1 1/4 cup soy milk

Sliced fruits, for topping

Vegan whipping cream, for topping

Directions:

Switch on the waffle maker and let it preheat.

Meanwhile, place flour in a bowl, stir in salt, baking powder, and sugar and whisk in whisk in remaining ingredients, except for topping, until incorporated.

Ladle the batter into the waffle maker and Cooking Time:

until firm and brown.

When done, top waffles with fruits and whipped cream and serve.

Nutrition:

Calories: 277 Cal

Fat: 8.3 g

Carbs: 42.5 g

Protein: 6.2 g

Fiber: 1.5 g

**Chickpea Omelet**

Preparation time: 5 minutes

Cooking time: 10 minutes

Servings: 1

Ingredients:

3 Tablespoon chickpea flour

1 small white onion, peeled, diced

½ teaspoon black salt

2 tablespoons chopped the dill

2 tablespoons chopped basil

1/8 teaspoon ground black pepper

2 Tablespoon olive oil

8 Tablespoon water

Directions:

Take a bowl, add flour in it along with salt and black pepper, stir until mixed, and then whisk in water until creamy.

Take a skillet pan, place it over medium heat, add 1 tablespoon oil and when hot, add onion and Cooking Time: for 4 minutes until cooked.

Add onion to omelet mixture and then stir until combined.

Add remaining oil into the pan, pour in prepared batter, spread evenly, and Cooking Time: for 3 minutes per side until cooked.

Serve omelet with bread.

Nutrition:

Calories: 150 Cal

Fat: 2 g

Carbs: 24.4 g

Protein: 10.2 g

Fiber: 5.8 g

## Scrambled Tofu Breakfast Burrito

Preparation time: 15 minutes

Cooking time: 20 minutes

Servings: 4

Ingredients:

For the Tofu:

12-ounce tofu, extra-firm, pressed

1/4 cup minced parsley

1 ½ teaspoon minced garlic

1 teaspoon nutritional yeast

1/4 teaspoon sea salt

1/2 teaspoon red chili powder

1/2 teaspoon cumin

1 teaspoon olive oil

1 Tablespoon hummus

For the Vegetables:

5 baby potatoes, chopped

1 medium red bell pepper, sliced

2 cups chopped kale

1/2 teaspoon ground cumin

1/8 teaspoon sea salt

1/2 teaspoon red chili powder

1 teaspoon oil

The Rest

4 large tortillas

1 medium avocado, chopped

Cilantro as needed

Salsa as needed

Directions:

Switch on the oven, then set it to 400 degrees F and let it preheat.

Take a baking sheet, add potato and bell pepper, drizzle with oil, season with all the spices, toss until coated and bake for 15 minutes until tender and nicely browned.

Then add kale to the potatoes, Cooking Time: for 5 minutes, and set aside until required.

In the meantime, take a skillet pan, place it over medium heat, add oil and when hot add tofu, crumble it well and Cooking Time: for 10 minutes until lightly browned.

In the meantime, take a small bowl, add hummus and remaining ingredients for the tofu and stir until combined.

Add hummus mixture into tofu, stir and Cooking Time: for 3 minutes, set aside until required.

Assemble the burritos and for this, distribute roasted vegetables on the tortilla, top with tofu, avocado, cilantro, and salsa, roll and then serve.

Nutrition:

Calories: 441 Cal

Fat: 19.6 g

Carbs: 53.5 g

Protein: 16.5 g

Fiber: 8 g

**Pancake**

Preparation time: 10 minutes

Cooking time: 18 minutes

Servings: 4

Ingredients:

Dry Ingredients:

1 cup buckwheat flour

1/8 teaspoon salt

½ teaspoon gluten-free baking powder

½ teaspoon baking soda

Wet Ingredients:

1 tablespoon almond butter

2 tablespoon maple syrup

1 tablespoon lime juice

1 cup coconut milk, unsweetened

Directions:

Take a medium bowl, add all the dry ingredients and stir until mixed.

Take another bowl, place all the wet ingredients, whisk until combined, and then gradually whisk in dry ingredients mixture until smooth and incorporated.

Take a frying pan, place it over medium heat, add 2 teaspoons oil and when hot, drop in batter and Cooking Time: for 3 minutes per side until cooked and lightly browned.

Serve pancakes and fruits and maple syrup.

Nutrition:

Calories: 148 Cal

Fat: 8.2 g

Carbs: 15 g

Protein: 4.6 g

Fiber: 1.7 g.

**Ginger and Greens Smoothie**

Preparation time: 5 minutes

Cooking time: 0 minute

Servings: 1

Ingredients:

1 frozen banana

2 cups baby spinach

2-inch piece of ginger, peeled, chopped

¼ teaspoon cinnamon

¼ teaspoon vanilla extract, unsweetened

1/8 teaspoon salt

1 scoop vanilla protein powder

1/8 teaspoon cayenne pepper

2 tablespoons lemon juice

1 cup of orange juice

Method:

Place all the ingredients in the order in a food processor or blender and then pulse for 2 to 3 minutes at high speed until smooth.

Pour the smoothie into a glass and then serve.

Nutrition Value:

Calories: 320 Cal

Fat: 7 g

Carbs: 64 g

Protein: 10 g

Fiber: 12 g

# *The Plant Based Lunch*

**Grilled Eggplant Roll-Ups**

Preparation Time: 5 min

Cooking Time: 8 min

servings: 8

Ingredients:

Olive oil, two tablespoons

Basil, fresh, chopped, two tablespoons

Onion, one half sliced paper-thin

Bell pepper, one half sliced paper-thin

Tomato, one large

Eggplant, one medium

Method:

After cutting off both of the ends of the eggplant, slice it into strips the long way that is about a quarter-inch thick.

Slice the onion, bell pepper, and the tomato very thinly and set to the side. Brush the olive oil onto the slices of eggplant and grill them in a skillet for three minutes on each side. When both sides are grilled, lay the slices of eggplant on a plate and lay a slice each of tomato, onion, and bell pepper on each zucchini slice. Sprinkle all with the black pepper and the basil. Carefully roll each slice as far as it will roll.

Nutrition: Calorie 59, 4 grams carbs, 3 grams protein, 3 grams fat

**Veggie Stuffed Peppers**

Preparation Time: 30 min

servings: 6

Ingredients:

Balsamic vinegar, two tablespoons

Parsley, fresh, one-quarter cup chopped

Scallions, one bunch, cleaned and sliced

Cucumber, one half, peeled and diced

Celery, washed and diced four stalks

Cherry tomatoes cut in quarters, one cup

Green bell peppers, three, cleaned and cut in half across the middle

Salt, one half teaspoon

Dijon mustard, three tablespoons

Black pepper, one teaspoon

Method:

In one bowl, mix together the mustard, rice wine vinegar, salt, and pepper. Add in the tomatoes, cucumbers, scallions, and celery and mix gently but well. Use a spoon to stuff this mix into the pepper halves.

Nutrition: Calories 117, 9 grams carbs, 7 grams protein, 3 grams fat

## Sprout Wraps

Preparation Time: 15 min

servings: 2

Ingredients:

Tortillas, whole-wheat , two large

Parsley, one-half cup chopped

Onion, green, two stalks

Black pepper, one teaspoon

Cucumber, one sliced thin

Bean sprouts, one cup

Salt, one half teaspoon

Lemon juice,  one tablespoon

Olive oil, one tablespoon

Method:

Lay out each of the tortilla wraps on a plate. Divide evenly all of the ingredients between the two tortillas, leaving about two inches on either side for rolling the tortilla up. When you have added all of the ingredients on the tortilla, then fold in the sides and roll the tortilla up into a cylinder shape.

Nutrition: Calories 226, 12 grams carbs, 10 grams protein, 3 grams fat

## Collard Wraps

Preparation Time: 20 min

servings: 4

Ingredients:

Wrap

Cherry tomatoes, four cut in half

Black olives, sliced, one quarter cup

Purple onion, one-half cup diced fine

Red bell pepper, one half of one cut in julienne strips

Cucumber, one medium-sized cut in julienne strips

Green collard leaves, four large

Sauce

Black pepper, one teaspoon

Salt, one half teaspoon

Dill, fresh, minced, two tablespoons

Cucumber, seeded and grated, one quarter cup

Olive oil, two tablespoons

White vinegar, one tablespoon

Garlic powder, one teaspoon

Method:

Place all of the ingredients on the list for the sauce in a mixing bowl and mix well. Store the dressing in the refrigerator. Wash off the collard leaves and dry them and then cut off the stem from each leaf. Cover each leaf with two tablespoons of the sauce you just made. In the middle of the collard leaf layer, all of the other ingredients. Fold the leaf up like a burrito by first folding the ends in and then rolling the leaf until it is all rolled. Cut into slices and serve with more dressing for dipping.

Nutrition per wrap: Calories 165, 7.36 grams carbs, 6.98 grams protein, 11.25 grams fat

**Grape Tomatoes and Spiral Zucchini**

Preparation Time: 5 min

Cooking Time: 10 min

servings: 2

Ingredients:

Zucchini, one large cut in spirals

Basil, fresh, chopped, one tablespoon

Black pepper, one teaspoon

Rosemary, one teaspoon

Salt, one half teaspoon

Lemon juice, one tablespoon

Crushed red pepper flakes, one quarter teaspoon

Grape tomatoes, one cup cut in half

Garlic, minced, two tablespoons

Olive oil, one tablespoon

Method:

Fry the minced garlic in the olive oil for one minute. Pour in the pepper, salt, red pepper flakes, and the tomatoes and mix well, then turn the heat lower. Simmer this mix for fifteen minutes. Add in the basil, rosemary, and the zucchini spiral noodles and turn the heat back up and Cooking Time: for two minutes, stirring constantly. Drizzle the lemon juice over all of it and serve.

Nutrition: Calories 117, 13 grams carbs, 4 grams protein, 5 grams fat

**Cauliflower Fried Rice**

Preparation Time: 5 min

Cooking Time: 10 min

servings: 4

Ingredients:

Riced cauliflower, twelve ounces frozen or fresh

Sesame oil, one tablespoon

Soy sauce, two tablespoons

Carrot, one-quarter cup chopped fine

Tofu, firm, cut into crumbles

Garlic, minced, two tablespoons

Green onion, one quarter cup

Method:

Cooking Time: the carrots and the riced cauliflower in the sesame oil for about five minutes, stirring sometimes. Stir in this mix the chopped green onion and the garlic and Cooking Time: for one minute. Add the tofu to the rice mix and stir about two to three minutes. Just before serving mix in the soy sauce.

Nutrition: Calories 114, 6 grams carbs, 4 grams protein, 8 grams fat

**Mediterranean Style Pasta**

Preparation Time: 10 min

Cooking Time: 15 min

servings: 4

Ingredients:

Whole-wheat pasta, twelve ounces cooked

Nutritional yeast, one quarter cup

Kalamata olives, ten, cut in half

Parsley, chopped, two tablespoons

Capers, two tablespoons

Tomatoes, diced, one half cup

Salt, one half teaspoon

Black pepper, one teaspoon

Garlic, minced, two tablespoons

Olive oil, two tablespoons

Spinach, one cup, packed

Method:

Fry together in the olive oil, the salt, spinach, and the pepper for ten minutes until the spinach wilts. Add in the capers, parsley, olives, and tomatoes and mix well, cooking for another five minutes. Blend in the whole-wheat pasta, sprinkle on the nutritional yeast, and serve immediately.

Nutrition: Calories 231, 6.5 grams carbs, 6.5 grams protein, 20 grams fat

**Squash and Sweet Potato Patties**

Preparation Time: 15 minutes

Cooking Time: 10 minutes

servings: 2

Ingredients:

Olive oil, two tablespoons

Salt, one half teaspoon

Black pepper, one teaspoon

Parsley, dried, one quarter teaspoon

Cumin, ground, one quarter teaspoon

Garlic powder, one half teaspoon

Sweet potato, cooked and mashed, two cups

Squash, shredded, one cup

Method:

Mix the sweet potato and squash in a mixing bowl. Add in all of the spices and mix these ingredients well. Heat the oil in a skillet and separate the mix into four equal portions. Drop the portions into the oil and flatten slightly with a fork. Fry each of the patties for five minutes on each side and serve.

Nutrition per patty: Calories 112, 6 grams carbs, 3 grams protein, 9 grams fat

**Stuffed Artichokes**

Preparation Time: 45 min

Cooking Time: 30 min

servings: 6

Ingredients:

Artichokes, three

Celery salt, one half teaspoon

Mushroom, chopped, one half cup

Salt, one half teaspoon

Black pepper, one teaspoon

Onion, minced, two tablespoons

Lemon juice, two tablespoons

Parsley, chopped, one tablespoon

Method:

Heat oven to 375. Tear off and discard the outside leaves of the artichokes. Cut the inside of the artichokes in half across the middle. Drop the halves into already boiling water and Cooking Time: them for twenty minutes. Mix together the seasonings, onions, mushrooms, lemon juice, chili sauce, and parsley and spoon this mixture into the boiled artichoke hearts. Place the filled hearts into a baking pan and bake for thirty minutes.

Nutrition: Calories 425, 17 grams carbs, 18 grams protein, 21 grams fat

**Lima Bean Casserole**

Preparation Time: 15 min

Cooking Time: 30 min

servings: 5

Ingredients:

Lima beans, canned two cups

Lemon juice, two teaspoons

Thyme, one half teaspoon

Black pepper, one teaspoon

Nutritional yeast, one half cup

Olive oil, two tablespoons

Dry mustard, two teaspoons

Salt, one half teaspoon

Cumin, one teaspoon

Method:

Heat oven to 375. Drain the beans and save the liquid. Dump the drained beans into an eight by eight-inch baking pan. Add the olive oil with the bean liquid to a skillet and heat until the warm. Add in the pepper, salt, cumin, thyme, dry mustard, and lemon juice and stir together well. Pour this mix over the beans in the baking pan and cover with the nutritional yeast. Bake for thirty minutes.

Nutrition: Calories 194, 19 grams carbs, 6 grams protein, 7 grams fat

**Corn and Okra Casserole**

Preparation Time: 20 min

Cooking Time: 30 min

servings: 6

Ingredients:

Okra, one pound

Garlic, one clove sliced

Parsley, chopped, one tablespoon

Olive oil, three tablespoons

Tomatoes, two large diced

Green bell pepper, one cleaned and sliced

Corn, whole kernel, one can

Onion, one small, sliced

Method:

Heat oven to 375. Cut the okra into bite-sized chunks. Cooking Time: the garlic, onion, okra, and green pepper in the olive oil for ten minutes. Stir in the parsley and the tomatoes and Cooking Time: for an additional ten minutes. Pour in the corn and dump the entire mixture into a nine by nine-inch baking pan and bake, not covered, for thirty minutes.

Nutrition: Calories 125, 17 grams carbs, 4 grams protein, 2 grams fat

**Cucumber Tomato Toast**

Preparation Time: 5 min

servings: 1

Ingredients:

Balsamic vinegar, one teaspoon

Oregano, dried, one half teaspoon

Cucumber, one half diced

Tomato, one half diced

Whole-grain flatbread, two slices

Salt one half teaspoon

Thyme, one quarter teaspoon

Black pepper, one half teaspoon

Olive oil, one teaspoon

Method:

Mix well the pepper, salt, olive oil, oregano, thyme, dill, tomato, and cucumber. Top the flatbread with the mix. Drizzle on vinegar to taste.

Nutrition info: Calories 177, 8 grams fat, 24 grams carbs, 3 grams protein

**Pasta Pomodoro with Olives and White Beans**

Preparation Time: 30 minutes

servings: 2

Ingredients:

Ziti or rigatoni, whole-wheat , four ounces

Nutritional yeast, one half cup

Cannellini beans, one fifteen ounce can drain and rinse

Black pepper, one half teaspoon

Basil, ground, one quarter cup

Black olives, two tablespoons chopped

Tomatoes, two medium-sized diced

Garlic, minced, two tablespoons

Olive oil, one tablespoon

Method:

Cooking Time: the pasta per the package instructions.
Cooking Time: the beans and garlic in the hot oil for five
minutes. Take the pan from the heat. Add in the olives,
pepper, basil, and tomatoes and mix well. Place the pasta
on two plates, evenly divided and top with the tomato

bean mix. Sprinkle on the nutritional yeast and serve.

Nutrition info: Calories 478, 16 grams fat, 14 grams fiber, 74 grams carbs, 21 grams protein

**Bean Bolognese**

Preparation Time: 40 minutes

servings: 4

Ingredients:

White beans, one fourteen ounce can drain and rinse

Fettuccini, whole-wheat , eight ounces

Onion, one small chop

Olive oil, two tablespoons

Parsley, fresh, chopped, one-quarter cup divided

Tomatoes, diced, one fourteen ounce can

Balsamic vinegar, one half cup

Celery, one quarter cup chop

Carrot, one half cup chop

Bay leaf, one

Garlic, minced, two tablespoons

Salt, one half teaspoon

Method:

Cooking Time: the pasta per the package directions. Cooking Time: carrot, onion, celery, and garlic in the oil for ten minutes. Add in the bay leaf and salt and stir for one minute. Throw away the bay leaf. Pour in the balsamic vinegar and boil for five minutes. Add in the beans, tomatoes, and two tablespoons of the parsley to the skillet and simmer for five minutes, stirring often. Spoon the pasta into four bowls. Top the pasta with the sauce mix from the skillet. Sprinkle on the remainder of the parsley and serve.

Nutrition info: Calories 442, 11 grams fat, 13 grams fiber, 68 grams carbs, 18 grams protein

**Fusilli with Tomatoes and Squash**

Preparation Time: 25 minutes

servings: 6

Ingredients:

Fusilli pasta, twelve ounces

Grape tomatoes, two cups, sliced in half

Black pepper, one half teaspoon

Rosemary, one half teaspoon

Squash, yellow, one pound

Onion, yellow, one thin slice

Salt, one half teaspoon

Thyme, chop, one tablespoon

Olive oil, two tablespoons

Method:

Cooking Time: the pasta per the package directions. Cut the neck off the squash. Cut the squash into quarters longwise and slice thin. Cooking Time: onion, pepper, squash, thyme, and salt in the hot olive oil for ten minutes, stirring often. Pour in the tomatoes and Cooking Time: for five more minutes. Add in the cooked pasta and mix well.

Nutrition info: Calories 311, 9 grams fat, 4 grams fiber, 49 grams carbs, 10 grams proteins

# *The Plant Based Dinner*

**Farro and Veggies**

Preparation Time: 15 minutes

Cooking Time: 40 minutes

servings: 4

Ingredients:

Farro and Veggies

Farro, two cups cooked

Olive oil, two tablespoons

Red bell pepper, one diced

Butter lettuce, one head, torn

Balsamic vinegar, two tablespoons

Dill, dried, one tablespoon

Black pepper, one teaspoon

Rosemary, one teaspoon

Salt, one half teaspoon

Red potatoes, one pound cut in wedges

Oregano, dried, one tablespoon

Paprika, one tablespoon

Garlic, minced, two tablespoons

Butter lettuce, one head torn

Red onion, cucumber, green and/or black olives for serving

Red Wine Vinaigrette

Olive oil, one quarter cup

Balsamic vinegar, three tablespoons

Lemon juice, two tablespoons

Oregano, dried, one tablespoon

Garlic, minced, one tablespoon

Red pepper flakes, crushed, one quarter teaspoon

Salt, one half teaspoon

Black pepper, one teaspoon

Method:

Heat oven to 425. Mix together well the garlic, paprika, rosemary, salt, pepper, oregano, dill, balsamic vinegar, and one tablespoon of the olive oil. Lay the bell peppers and potatoes in a nine by thirteen-inch baking dish and cover with the seasoning mixture you just assembled. Bake the veggies for forty-five minutes. While the veggies are baking blend together well all the vinaigrette ingredients. Divide the lettuce between four bowls and cover with the farro and add the roasted veggie mix. Drizzle the vinaigrette over the mix in the bowls and serve with olives, onion, and cucumber on the side.

Nutrition info: Calories 782, 3.8 grams fat, 19 grams carbs, 4.2 grams fiber

**Stuffed Eggplant**

Preparation Time: 10 min

Cooking Time: 40 min

servings: 4

Ingredients:

Eggplant, two medium-size cut in half

Quinoa, cooked, two cups

Mushrooms, button, one cup thin-slice

Red onion, one diced

Parsley, chopped fresh, three tablespoons for garnish

Salt, one half teaspoon

Black pepper, one teaspoon

Turmeric, one teaspoon

Thyme, dried, one tablespoon

Kale, two cups chopped

Lemon juice, one tablespoon

Lemon zest, one tablespoon

Garlic, powdered, one tablespoon

Olive oil, three tablespoons divided

Method:

Heat oven to 400. Use a spoon to scoop one-third of the eggplant flesh out; save it for another use. Use half of the olive oil to coat the halves of the eggplant and place them on a parchment paper-covered baking pan with the inside facing up. Use the rest of the olive oil for cooking the kale, garlic, mushrooms, onions, and quinoa for five minutes. Use lemon juice, lemon zest, pepper, salt, and thyme to season this mix. Use the mix to fill the eggplant halves and bake for twenty minutes. Sprinkle with parsley serve.

Nutrition info: Calories 339, 15 grams fat, 46 grams carbs, 12 grams protein

**Veggie Rice Skillet**

Preparation Time: 15 min

Cooking Time: 25 min

servings: four to six

Serve as dinner and take the leftovers to lunch the next day

Ingredients:

Parsley, fresh chopped, one third cup

Green olives, one cup

Vegetable broth, two and one half cups

Garlic, minced, two tablespoons

Olive oil, two tablespoons

Rosemary, one teaspoon

Marjoram, one teaspoon

Salt, one half teaspoon

Black pepper, one teaspoon

Oregano, dried, one teaspoon

Rice, brown or wild, one cup

Red onion, one half minced

Lemons, three

Method:

Add the onion and garlic to the olive oil and fry for five minutes. Pour in the broth, rice, and veggies and mix well and let this mixture boil. Let this simmer over a lowered heat for twenty to twenty-five minutes, or until the rice is cooked. Top the individual servings with fresh parsley, olives, and lemon slices.

Nutrition info: Calories 903, 55 grams fat, 54 grams carbs, 48 grams protein

**Brown Rice and Mushroom Risotto**

Preparation Time: 20 minutes

Cooking Time: 25 minutes

servings: 6

Ingredients:

Black pepper, one teaspoon

Salt, one half teaspoon

Parsley, dried, one tablespoon

Brown rice, four cups

Vegetable broth, two cups divided

Mushrooms, button, one cup, sliced thin

Shallot, one large, minced

Onion, one small, well diced

Garlic, minced, two tablespoons

Marjoram, one teaspoon

Olive oil, two tablespoons

Method:

Fry the shallot, onion, and garlic in the olive oil for five minutes. Pour in one cup of the vegetable's broth and the mushrooms, Cooking Time: for five more minutes. Into this mixture, add the other cup of the vegetable broth and the brown rice, cooking for ten minutes while stirring often. Pour in the salt, pepper, and parsley and turn the heat under the pot to low . Simmer this mixture for ten to fifteen minutes or until the rice is completely cooked.

Nutrition: Calories 297, 7.5 grams carbs, 7 grams protein, 26 grams fat

**Roast Baby Eggplant**

Preparation Time: 20 min

Cooking Time: 45 min

servings: 4

Ingredients:

To Cooking Time:

Baby eggplant, eight

Black pepper, one teaspoon

Olive oil, two tablespoons

Salt, one teaspoon

For Serving

Salt, one teaspoon

Olive oil, two tablespoons

Black pepper, one teaspoon

Nutritional yeast, one half cup

Method:

Heat oven to 350. Wipe off the eggplants and cut each one in half down the long way. Lay them on a baking pan with the inside up and coat the insides with olive oil and sprinkle on pepper and salt. Bake the baby eggplant for forty-five minutes or until they become soft and brown slightly. Just before you serve them, top each eggplant half with a teaspoon of the nutritional yeast and top that with the olive oil, pepper, and salt.

Nutrition per half an eggplant: Calories 44, 1 gram carbs, 1 gram protein, 4 grams fat


## Mediterranean Style Spaghetti Squash

Preparation Time: 20 min

servings: 2

Ingredients:

Baked spaghetti squash, two cups

Red onion, thin slice, one quarter cup

Olive oil, two tablespoons

Salt, one half teaspoon

Baby spinach, torn, one cup

Cherry tomatoes, six, cut in half

Garlic, minced, one teaspoon

Thyme, dried, one teaspoon

Rosemary, one teaspoon

Marjoram, one teaspoon

Chickpeas, one-third cup, rinse and drain

Parsley, fresh, chopped, one half cup

Method:

Fry the onion and the garlic in the olive oil for five minutes. Add in the tomatoes, rosemary, marjoram, thyme, and chickpeas and Cooking Time: three more minutes. Add in the salt, spinach, and spaghetti squash and Cooking Time: for five more minutes while stirring constantly. Sprinkle on the chopped parsley all over the top and serve.

Nutrition: Calories 272, 14 grams carbs, 11 grams protein, 10 grams fat

## Eggplant Casserole

Preparation Time: 5 min

Cooking Time: 30 min

servings: 6

Ingredients:

Eggplant, one medium

Tomato soup, one can

Rosemary, one teaspoon

Salt, one half teaspoon

Onion, chopped, one quarter cup

Celery, one-half cup chopped fine

Shallots, one-quarter cup chopped fine

Olive oil, two tablespoons

Method:

Heat oven to 375. Peel the eggplant and dice it into bite-sized cubes. Drop the cubes into boiling water and Cooking Time: them for five minutes, then drain them well. Put the eggplant in a nine by nine-inch baking pan. Fry the onion, celery, and shallots in the olive oil for five minutes. Pour in the soup and cook, stirring often, for five minutes. Pour this mixture over the eggplant in the baking dish and bake for thirty minutes.

Nutrition: Calories 267, 19 grams carbs, 13 grams protein, 9 grams fat


**Butternut Squash with Mustard Vinaigrette**

Preparation Time: 20 min

Cooking Time: 50 min

servings: 6

Ingredients:

Squash, three small butternuts peeled, seeded and cut in half

Shallots, eight, cut into wedges

Dry mustard, one tablespoon

Olive oil, four tablespoons

Salt, one half teaspoon

Turmeric, one teaspoon

Black pepper, one teaspoon

Balsamic vinegar, one tablespoon

Parsley, chopped, one quarter cup

Method:

Heat oven to 375. Use a large mixing bowl to mix the shallots and the squash with the salt, pepper, turmeric, and olive oil, tossing these to mix well and coat all of the pieces. Arrange the squash and shallots on a cookie sheet and bake them for fifty minutes. While the veggies are baking make vinaigrette with the balsamic vinegar, dry mustard, and the parsley. Arrange the baked veggies on a serving dish and drizzle the vinaigrette over them and serve.

Nutrition: Calories 135, 11 grams carbs, 1 gram protein, 10 grams fat

## Mini Black Bean Pitas

Preparation Time: 1 hour 10 minutes

Cooking Time: 30 min

servings: 8

Ingredients:

Black Beans

Black beans, canned drained and rinsed, two cups

Black pepper, one teaspoon

Lemon juice, two tablespoons

Lemon zest, one tablespoon

Coriander, ground, three quarters teaspoon

Cumin, ground, one teaspoon

Garlic powder, two teaspoons

Olive oil, one quarter cup

Paprika, smoked, one quarter teaspoon

Sauce

Tomatoes, two chopped

Dill, fresh, two tablespoons chopped

Garlic, minced, one tablespoon

Romaine lettuce, four leaves shred

Lemon juice, one tablespoon

Cucumber, one half thin sliced

Salt, one half teaspoon

Parsley, fresh, one quarter cup chop

Black pepper, one teaspoon

Red onion, one half thin sliced

Mini pita breads, sixteen

Method:

Mix coriander, cumin, pepper, lemon juice, lemon zest, paprika, garlic powder, and olive oil and pour over the black beans in a bowl. Let this rest in the refrigerator for one hour. In another bowl, mix dill, parsley, pepper, salt, garlic, and lemon juice. Refrigerate this mixture immediately. Place the black beans with the marinade in a skillet over medium-high heat and Cooking Time: until it boils. Let this mixture simmer over low heat until the liquid is cooked off, stirring frequently. Fill the pitas with the black beans and the sauce.

Nutrition info per wrap: Beans: Calories 154, 16 grams fat, 10 grams carbs. 9 grams protein/ Sauce: Calories 300, 5 grams fat, 56 grams carbs, 13 grams protein

**Pasta ala Erbe**

Preparation Time: 40 min

servings: 8

Ingredients:

Whole-wheat Fettucine, one pound

Tomato paste, two tablespoons

Hot water, one cup

Red pepper, crushed, one quarter teaspoon

Rosemary, one teaspoon

Salt, one half teaspoon

Garlic, four cloves peeled and sliced thin

Olive oil, six tablespoons divide

Leafy greens, such as beet/chard/spinach, 1.5 pounds chop (no stems)

Method:

Cooking Time: the pasta per the package instructions. Cooking Time: the garlic in four tablespoons of oil for two minutes. Toss in the greens a little at a time. As they cook, they will begin to wilt and will fit into the pan. Season with crushed pepper, rosemary, and salt and stir well. Cooking Time: this mixture for about ten minutes. Blend the water into the tomato paste. Add this to skillet and simmer for fifteen minutes. Add in the cooked pasta to the skillet mix and toss well.

Nutrition info: Calories 355, 14 grams fat, 9 grams fiber, 48 grams carbs, 13 grams protein

**Vegetarian Nachos**

Preparation Time: 15 minutes

servings: 6

Ingredients:

Oregano, dried, one tablespoon minced

Olive oil, two tablespoons

Hummus, one-third cup prepared

Red onion, two tablespoons minced

Black olives, two tablespoons chopped

Tofu, one-half cup cut into small crumbles

Black pepper, one half teaspoon

Lemon juice, one tablespoon

Grape tomatoes, one-half cup cut in quarters

Romaine lettuce, one cup chopped

Pita chips, whole-wheat , three cups

Nutritional yeast, one half cup

Method:

Blend together the lemon juice, oil, pepper, and hummus in a bowl. Spread a layer of the pita chips on a platter. Use a spoon to dribble three-fourths of the hummus mix over the chips. Garnish the chips with the olives, tomatoes, red onion, and lettuce. Spoon the remainder of the hummus decoratively in the middle and garnish with the nutritional yeast and the oregano.

Nutrition info one serving: Calories 159, 10 grams fat, 2 grams fiber, 13 grams carbs, 4 grams proteins


**Lasagna Zucchini Rolls**

Preparation Time: 45 min

Cooking Time: 30 min

servings: 4

Ingredients:

Zucchini, three large trimmed

Almonds, chopped, one quarter cup

Black pepper, one half teaspoon

Crushed red pepper, one quarter teaspoon

Garlic, minced, two teaspoons and two teaspoons

Italian seasoning, one teaspoon

Crushed tomatoes, two cups

Salt, one-quarter teaspoon and one quarter teaspoon

Olive oil, four tablespoons divided

Method:

Heat oven to 425. Spray oil a large cookie sheet. Cut slices from each zucchini down the length about one-quarter inch thick. Use three tablespoons of the olive oil to coat the strips and then sprinkle on one-quarter teaspoon of the salt. Bake the strips for twenty-five minutes until the zucchini strips are soft. Lower the oven temp to 350. In a bowl, mix the two teaspoons of the minced garlic, black pepper, crushed red pepper, Italian seasoning, and the tomatoes and mix well. Pour the tomato mix into a greased nine by thirteen-inch baking pan. Roll up each strip of zucchini and place it into the tomato mix in pan. Bake these for  thirty minutes. Garnish with the rest of the garlic and the chopped almonds.

Nutrition info per four rolls with sauce: Calories 324, 21 grams fat, 4 grams fiber, 19 grams carbs, 17 grams protein

**Sweet Potato and Black Bean Rice Bowl**

Preparation Time: 30 min

servings: 4

Ingredients:

Sweet chili sauce, two tablespoons

Black beans, one fifteen ounce can drain and rinse

Kale, fresh, four cups chopped

Red onion, one fine chop

Olive oil, three tablespoons

Water, one and one half cups

Sweet potato, two peeled and chopped into bite-sized pieces

Celery, one-half cup chopped

Garlic salt, one quarter teaspoon

Turmeric, one teaspoon

Oregano, one teaspoon

Long grain rice, three-fourths cup uncooked

Method:

Cooking Time: the rice in water with the garlic salt for twenty minutes. While the rice cooks put the sweet potato in the olive oil in a skillet and Cooking Time: for eight minutes, stirring often. Mix in the kale, celery, turmeric, oregano, onion, and beans and Cooking Time: for five more minutes. Stir in the chili sauce into the cooked rice and add to the potato mix; serve.

Nutrition info two cups: Calories 453, 8 grams fiber, 11 grams fat, 10 grams protein, 74 grams carbs

## Macaroni and Cheese

Preparation Time: 15 min

Cooking Time: 25 min

servings: 4

Ingredients:

Elbow macaroni, whole-grain , eight ounces

Apple cider vinegar, two teaspoons

Water, one cup (more if needed)

Red pepper, flakes, one eighth teaspoon

Salt, one half teaspoon

Dry mustard powder, one half teaspoon

Onion powder, one half teaspoon

Garlic powder, one half teaspoon

Garlic, minced, two tablespoons

Russet potato, peeled and grated, one cup (about two small potatoes)

Onion, yellow, chopped, one cup

Avocado oil, two tablespoons

Broccoli, one head with florets cut into bite-sized pieces

Nutritional yeast, one quarter cup

Method:

Cooking Time: the elbow pasta according to the directions on the package. When the pasta is almost done (with two or three minutes left), stir in the broccoli with the pasta. Drain the broccoli past mix and place it in a large bowl. During the time the pasta is cooking warm the olive oil in a saucepan over medium-high heat and Cooking Time: the salt and the onion for about five minutes. Stir in the onion powder, grated potato, garlic powder, mustard powder, and salt, garlic, and red pepper flakes. Mix this well and let it cooks for two minutes so the flavors will mix. Pour in the water and mix well. Continue stirring frequently while this mixture cooks for about eight to ten minutes until the potatoes are tender. Pour this mixture carefully into a blender with the vinegar and the nutritional yeast and blend carefully until it is smooth and creamy. Pour this mix over the past in the large bowl, mix well, and serve.

Nutrition: Calories 506. 21.7 grams fat, 66.5 grams carbs, 8.7 grams fiber, 18.3 grams protein

**Avocado, Kale, and Black Bean Bowl**

Preparation Time: 20 min

Cooking Time: 30 min

servings: 4

Ingredients:

Kale, one bunch with ribs removed and chopped into bite-sized pieces

Cherry tomatoes, cut in half, one half cup

Cayenne pepper, one quarter teaspoon

Chili powder, one quarter teaspoon

Garlic, minced, two tablespoons

Shallot, one chopped finely

Black beans, two fifteen ounce cans drained and rinsed

Lime juice, one quarter cup

Cilantro, chopped, one half cup

Salsa Verde, mild, one half cup

Avocado, one, peeled, pitted, cut into big chunks

Cumin, one half teaspoon

Jalapeno, one half, seeded and chopped finely

Olive oil, two tablespoons

Salt, one quarter teaspoon

Brown rice, one cup rinsed

Method:

Cooking Time: the rice per the package instructions and then let it rest for fifteen minutes and then salt the rice and fluff it with a fork. While the rice is cooking, make the kale salad by blending together the cumin, salt, olive oil, jalapeno, and the lime juice and then put in the chopped kale. In another bowl, mix together well the cilantro, lime juice, Salsa Verde, and the chunks of the avocado. Place the beans in a saucepan and warm them over low heat in one tablespoon of olive oil. Mix in the shallot and the garlic and Cooking Time: for three minutes, then stir in the chili powder and cayenne pepper. Cooking Time: for seven to ten minutes. For serving, add the kale salad with the rice and the bean mixture to bowls and add in some of the Salsa Verde avocado. Toss chopped cherry tomatoes on top for garnish.

Nutrition: Calories 424, 12 grams fat, 57 grams carbs, 12 grams fiber, 24 grams protein

# The Plant Based Snacks for Morning and Afternoon

**Black Bean Lime Dip**

Preparation time: 5 minutes

Cooking time: 6 minutes

Servings: 4

Ingredients:

15.5 ounces cooked black beans

1 teaspoon minced garlic

½ of a lime, juiced

1 inch of ginger, grated

1/3 teaspoon salt

1/3 teaspoon ground black pepper

1 tablespoon olive oil

Method:

Take a frying pan, add oil and when hot, add garlic and ginger and Cooking Time: for 1 minute until fragrant.

Then add beans, splash with some water and fry for 3 minutes until hot.

Season beans with salt and black pepper, drizzle with lime juice, then remove the pan from heat and mash the beans until smooth pasta comes together.

Serve the dip with whole-grain bread sticks or vegetables.

Nutrition Value:

Calories: 374 Cal

Fat: 14 g

Carbs: 46 g

Protein: 15 g

Fiber: 17 g

**Beetroot Hummus**

Preparation time: 10 minutes

Cooking time: 60 minutes

Servings: 4

Ingredients:

15 ounces cooked chickpeas

3 small beets

1 teaspoon minced garlic

1/2 teaspoon smoked paprika

1 teaspoon of sea salt

1/4 teaspoon red chili flakes

2 tablespoons olive oil

1 lemon, juiced

2 tablespoon tahini

1 tablespoon chopped almonds

1 tablespoon chopped cilantro

Method:

Drizzle oil over beets, season with salt, then wrap beets in a foil and bake for 60 minutes at 425 degrees F until tender.

When done, let beet cool for 10 minutes, then peel and dice them and place them in a food processor.

Add remaining ingredients and pulse for 2 minutes until smooth, tip the hummus in a bowl, drizzle with some more oil, and then serve straight away.

Nutrition Value:

Calories: 50.1 Cal

Fat: 2.5 g

Carbs: 5 g

Protein: 2 g

Fiber: 1 g

**Zucchini Hummus**

Preparation time: 5 minutes

Cooking time: 0 minute

Servings: 8

Ingredients:

1 cup diced zucchini

1/2 teaspoon sea salt

1 teaspoon minced garlic

2 teaspoons ground cumin

3 tablespoons lemon juice

1/3 cup tahini

Method:

Place all the ingredients in a food processor and pulse for 2 minutes until smooth.

Tip the hummus in a bowl, drizzle with oil and serve.

Nutrition Value:

Calories: 65 Cal

Fat: 5 g

Carbs: 3 g

Protein: 2 g

Fiber: 1 g

## Chipotle and Lime Tortilla Chips

Preparation time: 10 minutes

Cooking time: 15 minutes

Servings: 4

Ingredients:

12 ounces whole-wheat tortillas

4 tablespoons chipotle seasoning

1 tablespoon olive oil

4 limes, juiced

Method:

Whisk together oil and lime juice, brush it well on tortillas, then sprinkle with chipotle seasoning and bake for 15 minutes at 350 degrees F until crispy, turning halfway.

When done, let the tortilla cool for 10 minutes, then break it into chips and serve.

Nutrition Value:

Calories: 150 Cal

Fat: 7 g

Carbs: 18 g

Protein: 2 g

Fiber: 2 g

**Carrot and Sweet Potato Fritters**

Preparation time: 10 minutes

Cooking time: 8 minutes

Servings: 10

Ingredients:

1/3 cup quinoa flour

1½ cups shredded sweet potato

1 cup grated carrot

1/3 teaspoon ground black pepper

2/3 teaspoon salt

2 teaspoons curry powder

2 flax eggs

2 tablespoons coconut oil

Method:

Place all the ingredients in a bowl, except for oil, stir well until combined and then shape the mixture into ten small patties

Take a large pan, place it over medium-high heat, add oil and when it melts, add patties in it and Cooking Time: for 3 minutes per side until browned.

Serve straight away

Nutrition Value:

Calories: 70 Cal

Fat: 3 g

Carbs: 8 g

Protein: 1 g

Fiber: 1 g

**Tomato and Pesto Toast**

Preparation time: 5 minutes

Cooking time: 0 minute

Servings: 4

Ingredients:

1 small tomato, sliced

¼ teaspoon ground black pepper

1 tablespoon vegan pesto

2 tablespoons hummus

1 slice of whole-grain bread, toasted

Hemp seeds as needed for garnishing

Method:

Spread hummus on one side of the toast, top with tomato slices and then drizzle with pesto.

Sprinkle black pepper on the toast along with hemp seeds and then serve straight away.

Nutrition Value:

Calories: 214 Cal

Fat: 7.2 g

Carbs: 32 g

Protein: 6.5 g

Fiber: 3 g

**Avocado and Sprout Toast**

Preparation time: 5 minutes

Cooking time: 0 minute

Servings: 4

Ingredients:

1/2 of a medium avocado, sliced

1 slice of whole-grain bread, toasted

2 tablespoons sprouts

2 tablespoons hummus

¼ teaspoon lemon zest

½ teaspoon hemp seeds

¼ teaspoon red pepper flakes

Method:

Spread hummus on one side of the toast and then top with avocado slices and sprouts.

Sprinkle with lemon zest, hemp seeds, and red pepper flakes and then serve straight away.

Nutrition Value:

Calories: 200 Cal

Fat: 10.5 g

Carbs: 22 g

Protein: 7 g

Fiber: 7 g


**Apple and Honey Toast**

Preparation time: 5 minutes

Cooking time: 0 minute

Servings: 4

Ingredients:

½ of a small apple, cored, sliced

1 slice of whole-grain bread, toasted

1 tablespoon honey

2 tablespoons hummus

1/8 teaspoon cinnamon

Method:

Spread hummus on one side of the toast, top with apple slices and then drizzle with honey.

Sprinkle cinnamon on it and then serve straight away.

Nutrition Value:

Calories: 212 Cal

Fat: 7 g

Carbs: 35 g

Protein: 4 g

Fiber: 5.5 g

## Zucchini Fritters

Preparation time: 10 minutes

Cooking time: 6 minutes

Servings: 12

Ingredients:

1/2 cup quinoa flour

3 1/2 cups shredded zucchini

1/2 cup chopped scallions

1/3 teaspoon ground black pepper

1 teaspoon salt

2 tablespoons coconut oil

2 flax eggs

Method:

Squeeze moisture from the zucchini by wrapping it in a cheesecloth and then transfer it to a bowl.

Add remaining ingredients, except for oil, stir until combined and then shape the mixture into twelve patties.

Take a skillet pan, place it over medium-high heat, add oil and when hot, add patties and Cooking Time: for 3 minutes per side until brown.

Serve the patties with favorite vegan sauce.

Nutrition Value:

Calories: 37 Cal

Fat: 1 g

Carbs: 4 g

Protein: 2 g

Fiber: 1 g

## Zucchini Chips

Preparation time: 10 minutes

Cooking time: 120 minutes

Servings: 4

Ingredients:

1 large zucchini, thinly sliced

1 teaspoon salt

2 tablespoons olive oil

Method:

Pat dry zucchini slices and then spread them in an even layer on a baking sheet lined with parchment sheet.

Whisk together salt and oil, brush this mixture over zucchini slices on both sides and then bake for 2 hours or more until brown and crispy.

When done, let the chips cool for 10 minutes and then serve straight away.

Nutrition Value:

Calories: 54 Cal

Fat: 5 g

Carbs: 1 g

Protein: 0 g

Fiber: 0.3 g


**Rosemary Beet Chips**

Preparation time: 10 minutes

Cooking time: 20 minutes

Servings: 3

Ingredients:

3 large beets, scrubbed, thinly sliced

1/8 teaspoon ground black pepper

¼ teaspoon of sea salt

3 sprigs of rosemary, leaves chopped

4 tablespoons olive oil

Method:

Spread beet slices in a single layer between two large baking sheets, brush the slices with oil, then season with spices and rosemary, toss until well coated, and bake for 20 minutes at 375 degrees F until crispy, turning halfway.

When done, let the chips cool for 10 minutes and then serve.

Nutrition Value:

Calories: 79 Cal

Fat: 4.7 g

Carbs: 8.6 g

Protein: 1.5 g

Fiber: 2.5 g

## Quinoa Broccoli Tots

Preparation time: 10 minutes

Cooking time: 20 minutes

Servings: 16

Ingredients:

2 tablespoons quinoa flour

2 cups steamed and chopped broccoli florets

1/2 cup nutritional yeast

1 teaspoon garlic powder

1 teaspoon miso paste

2 flax eggs

2 tablespoons hummus

Method:

Place all the ingredients in a bowl, stir until well combined, and then shape the mixture into sixteen small balls.

Arrange the balls on a baking sheet lined with parchment paper, spray with oil and bake at 400 degrees F for 20 minutes until brown, turning halfway.

When done, let the tots cool for 10 minutes and then serve straight away.

Nutrition Value:

Calories: 19 Cal

Fat: 0 g

Carbs: 2 g

Protein: 1 g

Fiber: 0.5 g

**Spicy Roasted Chickpeas**

Preparation time: 10 minutes

Cooking time: 20 minutes

Servings: 6

Ingredients:

30 ounces cooked chickpeas

½ teaspoon salt

2 teaspoons mustard powder

½ teaspoon cayenne pepper

2 tablespoons olive oil

Method:

Place all the ingredients in a bowl and stir until well coated and then spread the chickpeas in an even layer on a baking sheet greased with oil.

Bake the chickpeas for 20 minutes at 400 degrees F until

golden brown and crispy and then serve straight away.

Nutrition Value:

Calories: 187.1 Cal

Fat: 7.4 g

Carbs: 24.2 g

Protein: 7.3 g

Fiber: 6.3 g


**Nacho Kale Chips**

Preparation time: 10 minutes

Cooking time: 14 hours

Servings: 10

Ingredients:

2 bunches of curly kale

2 cups cashews, soaked, drained

1/2 cup chopped red bell pepper

1 teaspoon garlic powder

1 teaspoon salt

2 tablespoons red chili powder

1/2 teaspoon smoked paprika

1/2 cup nutritional yeast

1 teaspoon cayenne

3 tablespoons lemon juice

3/4 cup water

Method:

Place all the ingredients except for kale in a food processor and pulse for 2 minutes until smooth.

Place kale in a large bowl, pour in the blended mixture, mix until coated, and dehydrate for 14 hours at 120 degrees F until crispy.

If dehydrator is not available, spread kale between two baking sheets and bake for 90 minutes at 225 degrees F until crispy, flipping halfway.

When done, let chips cool for 15 minutes and then serve.

Nutrition Value:

Calories: 191 Cal

Fat: 12 g

Carbs: 16 g

Protein: 9 g

Fiber: 2 g

**Red Salsa**

Preparation time: 10 minutes

Cooking time: 0 minute

Servings: 8

Ingredients:

30 ounces diced fire-roasted tomatoes

4 tablespoons diced green chilies

1 medium jalapeño pepper, deseeded

1/2 cup chopped green onion

1 cup chopped cilantro

1 teaspoon minced garlic

½ teaspoon of sea salt

1 teaspoon ground cumin

¼ teaspoon stevia

3 tablespoons lime juice

Method:

Place all the ingredients in a food processor and process for 2 minutes until smooth.

Tip the salsa in a bowl, taste to adjust seasoning and then serve.

Nutrition Value:

Calories: 71 Cal

Fat: 0.2 g

Carbs: 19 g

Protein: 2 g

Fiber: 4.1 g

**Tomato Hummus**

Preparation time: 5 minutes

Cooking time: 0 minute

Servings: 4

Ingredients:

1/4 cup sun-dried tomatoes, without oil

1 ½ cups cooked chickpeas

1 teaspoon minced garlic

1/2 teaspoon salt

2 tablespoons sesame oil

1 tablespoon lemon juice

1 tablespoon olive oil

1/4 cup of water

Method:

Place all the ingredients in a food processor and process for 2 minutes until smooth.

Tip the hummus in a bowl, drizzle with more oil, and then serve straight away.

Nutrition Value:

Calories: 122.7 Cal

Fat: 4.1 g

Carbs: 17.8 g

Protein: 5.1 g

Fiber: 3.5 g

## Marinated Mushrooms

Preparation time: 10 minutes

Cooking time: 7 minutes

Servings: 6

Ingredients:

12 ounces small button mushrooms

1 teaspoon minced garlic

1/4 teaspoon dried thyme

1/2 teaspoon sea salt

1/2 teaspoon dried basil

1/2 teaspoon red pepper flakes

1/4 teaspoon dried oregano

1/2 teaspoon maple syrup

1/4 cup apple cider vinegar

1/4 cup and 1 teaspoon olive oil

2 tablespoons chopped parsley

Method:

Take a skillet pan, place it over medium-high heat, add 1 teaspoon oil and when hot, add mushrooms and Cooking Time: for 5 minutes until golden brown.

Meanwhile, prepare the marinade and for this, place remaining ingredients in a bowl and whisk until combined.

When mushrooms have cooked, transfer them into the bowl of marinade and toss until well coated.

Serve straight away

Nutrition Value:

Calories: 103 Cal

Fat: 9 g

Carbs: 2 g

Protein: 1 g

Fiber: 1 g

**Hummus Quesadillas**

Preparation time: 5 minutes

Cooking time: 15 minutes

Servings: 1

Ingredients:

1 tortilla, whole wheat

1/4 cup diced roasted red peppers

1 cup baby spinach

1/3 teaspoon minced garlic

¼ teaspoon salt

¼ teaspoon ground black pepper

1/4 teaspoon olive oil

1/4 cup hummus

Oil as needed

Method:

Place a large pan over medium heat, add oil and when hot, add red peppers and garlic, season with salt and black pepper and Cooking Time: for 3 minutes until sauté.

Then stir in spinach, Cooking Time: for 1 minute, remove the pan from heat and transfer the mixture in a bowl.

Prepare quesadilla and for this, spread hummus on one-half of the tortilla, then spread spinach mixture on it, cover the filling with the other half of the tortilla and Cooking Time: in a pan for 3 minutes per side until browned.

When done, cut the quesadilla into wedges and serve.

Nutrition Value:

Calories: 187 Cal

Fat: 9 g

Carbs: 16.3 g

Protein: 10.4 g

Fiber: 0 g

**Nacho Cheese Sauce**

Preparation time: 5 minutes

Cooking time: 10 minutes

Servings: 4

Ingredients:

3 tablespoons flour

1/4 teaspoon garlic salt

1/4 teaspoon salt

1/2 teaspoon cumin

1/4 teaspoon paprika

1 teaspoon red chili powder

1/8 teaspoon cayenne powder

1 cup vegan cashew yogurt

1 1/4 cups vegetable broth

Method:

Take a small saucepan, place it over medium heat, pour in vegetable broth, and bring it to a boil.

Then whisk together flour and yogurt, add to the boiling broth, stir in all the spices, switch heat to medium-low level and Cooking Time: for 5 minutes until thickened.

Serve straight away.

Nutrition Value:

Calories: 282 Cal

Fat: 1 g

Carbs: 63 g

Protein: 3 g

Fiber: 12 g

## Avocado Tomato Bruschetta

Preparation time: 10 minutes

Cooking time: 0 minute

Servings: 4

Ingredients:

3 slices of whole-grain bread

6 chopped cherry tomatoes

½ of sliced avocado

½ teaspoon minced garlic

½ teaspoon ground black pepper

2 tablespoons chopped basil

½ teaspoon of sea salt

1 teaspoon balsamic vinegar

Method:

Place tomatoes in a bowl, and then stir in vinegar until mixed.

Top bread slices with avocado slices, then top evenly with tomato mixture, garlic and basil, and season with salt and black pepper.

Serve straight away

Nutrition Value:

Calories: 131 Cal

Fat: 7.3 g

Carbs: 15 g

Protein: 2.8 g

Fiber: 3.2 g


## Cinnamon Bananas

Preparation time: 5 minutes

Cooking time: 8 minutes

Servings: 2

Ingredients:

2 bananas, peeled, sliced

1 teaspoon cinnamon

2 tablespoons granulated Splenda

1/4 teaspoon nutmeg

Method:

Prepare the cinnamon mixture and for this, place all the ingredients in a bowl, except for banana, and stir until mixed.

Take a large skillet pan, place it over medium heat, spray with oil, add banana slices and sprinkle with half of the prepared cinnamon mixture.

Cooking Time: for 3 minutes, then sprinkle with remaining prepared cinnamon mixture and continue cooking for 3 minutes until tender and hot.

Serve straight away.

Nutrition Value:

Calories: 155 Cal

Fat: 2 g

Carbs: 39 g

Protein: 1 g

Fiber: 3 g

# *The Plant-based Desserts*

**Key Lime Pie**

Preparation time: 3 hours and 15 minutes

Cooking time: 0 minute

Servings: 12

Ingredients:

For the Crust:

¾ cup coconut flakes, unsweetened

1 cup dates, soaked in warm water for 10 minutes in water, drained

For the Filling:

¾ cup of coconut meat

1 ½ avocado, peeled, pitted

2 tablespoons key lime juice

¼ cup agave

Directions:

Prepare the crust, and for this, place all its ingredients in a food processor and pulse for 3 to 5 minutes until the thick paste comes together.

Take an 8-inch pie pan, grease it with oil, pour crust mixture in it and spread and press the mixture evenly in the bottom and along the sides, and freeze until required.

Prepare the filling and for this, place all its ingredients in a food processor, and pulse for 2 minutes until smooth.

Pour the filling into prepared pan, smooth the top, and freeze for 3 hours until set.

Cut pie into slices and then serve.

Nutrition:

Calories: 213 Cal

Fat: 10 g

Carbs: 29 g

Protein: 1200 g

Fiber: 6 g

## Chocolate Mint Grasshopper Pie

Preparation time: 4 hours and 15 minutes

Cooking time: 0 minute

Servings: 4

Ingredients:

For the Crust:

1 cup dates, soaked in warm water for 10 minutes in water, drained

1/8 teaspoons salt

1/2 cup pecans

1 teaspoons cinnamon

1/2 cup walnuts

For the Filling:

½ cup mint leaves

2 cups of cashews, soaked in warm water for 10 minutes

in water, drained

2 tablespoons coconut oil

1/4 cup and 2 tablespoons of agave

1/4 teaspoons spirulina

1/4 cup water

Directions:

Prepare the crust, and for this, place all its ingredients in a food processor and pulse for 3 to 5 minutes until the thick paste comes together.

Take a 6-inch springform pan, grease it with oil, place crust mixture in it and spread and press the mixture evenly in the bottom and along the sides, and freeze until required.

Prepare the filling and for this, place all its ingredients in a food processor, and pulse for 2 minutes until smooth.

Pour the filling into prepared pan, smooth the top, and freeze for 4 hours until set.

Cut pie into slices and then serve.

Nutrition:

Calories: 223.7 Cal

Fat: 7.5 g

Carbs: 36 g

Protein: 2.5 g

Fiber: 1 g

## Peanut Butter Energy Bars

Preparation time: 5 hours and 15 minutes

Cooking time: 5 minutes

Servings: 16

Ingredients:

1/2 cup cranberries

12 Medjool dates, pitted

1 cup roasted almond

1 tablespoon chia seeds

1 1/2 cups oats

1/8 teaspoon salt

1/4 cup and 1 tablespoon agave nectar

1/2 teaspoon vanilla extract, unsweetened

1/3 cup and 1 tablespoon peanut butter, unsalted

2 tablespoons water

Directions:

Place an almond in a food processor, pulse until chopped, and then transfer into a large bowl.

Add dates into the food processor along with oats, pour in water, and pulse for dates are chopped.

Add dates mixture into the almond mixture, add chia seeds and berries and stir until mixed.

Take a saucepan, place it over medium heat, add remaining butter and remaining ingredients, stir and Cooking Time: for 5 minutes until mixture reaches to a liquid consistency.

Pour the butter mixture over date mixture, and then stir until well combined.

Take an 8 by 8 inches baking tray, line it with parchment sheet, add date mixture in it, spread and press it evenly and refrigerate for 5 hours.

Cut it into sixteen bars and serve.

Nutrition:

Calories: 187 Cal

Fat: 7.5 g

Carbs: 27.2 g

Protein: 4.7 g

Fiber: 2 g

**Black Bean Brownie Pops**

Preparation time: 45 minutes

Cooking time: 2 minutes

Servings: 12

Ingredients:

3/4 cup chocolate chips

15 ounce cooked black beans

1 tablespoon maple syrup

5 tablespoons cacao powder

1/8 teaspoon sea salt

2 tablespoons sunflower seed butter

Directions:

Place black beans in a food processor, add remaining ingredients, except for chocolate, and pulse for 2 minutes until combined and the dough starts to come together.

Shape the dough into twelve balls, arrange them on a baking sheet lined with parchment paper, then insert a toothpick into each ball and refrigerate for 20 minutes.

Then meat chocolate in the microwave for 2 minutes, and dip brownie pops in it until covered.

Return the pops into the refrigerator for 10 minutes until

set and then serve.

Nutrition:

Calories: 130 Cal

Fat: 6 g

Carbs: 17 g

Protein: 4 g

Fiber: 1 g

## Lemon Cashew Tart

Preparation time: 3 hours and 15 minutes

Cooking time: 0 minute

Servings: 12

Ingredients:

For the Crust:

1 cup almonds

4 dates, pitted, soaked in warm water for 10 minutes in water, drained

1/8 teaspoon crystal salt

1 teaspoon vanilla extract, unsweetened

For the Cream:

1 cup cashews, soaked in warm water for 10 minutes in water, drained

1/4 cup water

1/4 cup coconut nectar

1 teaspoon coconut oil

1 teaspoon vanilla extract, unsweetened

1 lemon, Juiced

1/8 teaspoon crystal salt

For the Topping:

Shredded coconut as needed

Directions:

Prepare the cream and for this, place all its ingredients in a food processor, pulse for 2 minutes until smooth, and then refrigerate for 1 hour.

Then prepare the crust, and for this, place all its ingredients in a food processor and pulse for 3 to 5 minutes until the thick paste comes together.

Take a tart pan, grease it with oil, place crust mixture in it and spread and press the mixture evenly in the bottom and along the sides, and freeze until required.

Pour the filling into the prepared tart, smooth the top, and refrigerate for 2 hours until set.

Cut tart into slices and then serve.

Nutrition:

Calories: 166 Cal

Fat: 10 g

Carbs: 15 g

Protein: 5 g

Fiber: 1 g

**Peppermint Oreos**

Preparation time: 2 hours

Cooking time: 0 minute

Servings: 12

Ingredients:

For the Cookies:

1 cup dates

2/3 cup brazil nuts

3 tablespoons carob powder

2/3 cup almonds

1/8 teaspoon sea salt

3 tablespoons water

For the Crème:

2 tablespoons almond butter

1 cup coconut chips

2 tablespoons melted coconut oil

1 cup coconut shreds

3 drops of peppermint oil

1/2 teaspoon vanilla powder

For the Dark Chocolate:

3/4 cup cacao powder

1/2 cup date paste

1/3 cup coconut oil, melted

Directions:

Prepare the cookies, and for this, place all its ingredients in a food processor and pulse for 3 to 5 minutes until the dough comes together.

Then place the dough between two parchment sheets, roll the dough, then cut out twenty-four cookies of the desired shape and freeze until solid.

Prepare the crème, and for this, place all its ingredients in a food processor and pulse for 2 minutes until smooth.

When cookies have harden, sandwich crème in between

the cookies by placing dollops on top of a cookie and then pressing it with another cookie.

Freeze the cookies for 30 minutes and in the meantime, prepare chocolate and for this, place all its ingredients in a bowl and whisk until combined.

Dip frouncesen cookie sandwich into chocolate, at least two times, and then freeze for another 30 minutes until chocolate has hardened.

Serve straight away.

Nutrition:

Calories: 470 Cal

Fat: 32 g

Carbs: 51 g

Protein: 7 g

Fiber: 12 g

**Snickers Pie**

Preparation time: 4 hours

Cooking time: 0 minute

Servings: 16

Ingredients:

For the Crust:

12 Medjool dates, pitted

1 cup dried coconut, unsweetened

5 tablespoons cocoa powder

1/2 teaspoon sea salt

1 teaspoon vanilla extract, unsweetened

1 cup almonds

For the Caramel Layer:

10 Medjool dates, pitted, soaked for 10 minutes in warm water, drained

2 teaspoons vanilla extract, unsweetened

3 teaspoons coconut oil

3 tablespoons almond butter, unsalted

For the Peanut Butter Mousse:

3/4 cup peanut butter

2 tablespoons maple syrup

1/2 teaspoon vanilla extract, unsweetened

1/8 teaspoon sea salt

28 ounces coconut milk, chilled

Directions:

Prepare the crust, and for this, place all its ingredients in a food processor and pulse for 3 to 5 minutes until the thick paste comes together.

Take a baking pan, line it with parchment paper, place crust mixture in it and spread and press the mixture evenly in the bottom, and freeze until required.

Prepare the caramel layer, and for this, place all its ingredients in a food processor and pulse for 2 minutes until smooth.

Pour the caramel on top of the prepared crust, smooth the top and freeze for 30 minutes until set.

Prepare the mousse and for this, separate coconut milk and its solid, then add solid from coconut milk into a food processor, add remaining ingredients and then pulse for 1 minute until smooth.

Top prepared mousse over caramel layer, and then freeze for 3 hours until set.

Serve straight away.

Nutrition:

Calories: 456 Cal

Fat: 33 g

Carbs: 37 g

Protein: 8.3 g

Fiber: 5 g


**Double Chocolate Orange Cheesecake**

Preparation time: 4 hours

Cooking time: 0 minute

Servings: 12

Ingredients:

For the Base:

9 Medjool dates, pitted

1/3 cup Brazil nuts

2 tablespoons maple syrup

1/3 cup walnuts

2 tablespoons water

3 tablespoons cacao powder

For the Chocolate Cheesecake:

1/2 cup cacao powder

1 1/2 cups cashews, soaked for 10 minutes in warm water, drained

1/3 cup liquid coconut oil

1 teaspoon vanilla extract, unsweetened

1/3 cup maple syrup

1/3 cup water

For the Orange Cheesecake:

2 oranges, juiced

1/4 cup maple syrup

1 cup cashews, soaked for 10 minutes in warm water, drained

1 teaspoon vanilla extract, unsweetened

2 tablespoons coconut butter

1/2 cup liquid coconut oil

2 oranges, zested

4 drops of orange essential oil

For the Chocolate Topping:

3 tablespoons cacao powder

3 drops of orange essential oil

2 tablespoons liquid coconut oil

3 tablespoons maple syrup

Directions:

Prepare the base, and for this, place all its ingredients in a food processor and pulse for 3 to 5 minutes until the thick paste comes together.

Take a cake tin, place crust mixture in it and spread and press the mixture evenly in the bottom, and freeze until required.

Prepare the chocolate cheesecake, and for this, place all its ingredients in a food processor and pulse for 2 minutes until smooth.

Pour the chocolate cheesecake mixture on top of the prepared base, smooth the top and freeze for 20 minutes until set.

Then prepare the orange cheesecake and for this, place all its ingredients in a food processor, and pulse for 2 minutes until smooth

Top orange cheesecake mixture over chocolate

cheesecake, and then freeze for 3 hours until hardened.

Then prepare the chocolate topping and for this, take a bowl, add all the ingredients in it and stir until well combined.

Spread chocolate topping over the top, freeze the cake for 10 minutes until the topping has hardened and then slice to serve.

Nutrition:

Calories: 508 Cal

Fat: 34.4 g

Carbs: 44 g

Protein: 8 g

Fiber: 3 g

**Coconut Ice Cream Cheesecake**

Preparation time: 3 hours

Cooking time: 0 minute

Servings: 4

Ingredients:

For the First Layer:

1 cup mixed nuts

3/4 cup dates, soaked for 10 minutes in warm water

2 tablespoons almond milk

For the Second Layer:

1 medium avocado, diced

1 cup cashew nuts, soaked for 10 minutes in warm water

3 cups strawberries, sliced

1 tablespoon chia seeds, soaked in 3 tablespoons soy milk

1/2 cup agave

1 cup melted coconut oil

1/2 cup shredded coconut

1 lime, juiced

Directions:

Prepare the first layer, and for this, place all its ingredients in a food processor and pulse for 3 to 5 minutes until the thick paste comes together.

Take a springform pan, place crust mixture in it and spread and press the mixture evenly in the bottom, and freeze until required.

Prepare the second layer, and for this, place all its ingredients in a food processor and pulse for 2 minutes until smooth.

Pour the second layer on top of the first layer, smooth the top, and freeze for 4 hours until hard.

Serve straight away.

Nutrition:

Calories: 411.3 Cal

Fat: 30.8 g

Carbs: 28.7 g

Protein: 4.7 g

Fiber: 1.3 g

**Matcha Coconut Cream Pie**

Preparation time: 5 minutes

Cooking time: 0 minute

Servings: 4

Ingredients:

For the Crust:

1/2 cup ground flaxseed

3/4 cup shredded dried coconut

1 cup Medjool dates, pitted

3/4 cup dehydrated buckwheat groats

1/4 teaspoons sea salt

For the Filling:

1 cup dried coconut flakes

4 cups of coconut meat

1/4 cup and 2 Tablespoons coconut nectar

1/2 Tablespoons vanilla extract, unsweetened

1/4 teaspoons sea salt

2/3 cup and 2 Tablespoons coconut butter

1 Tablespoons matcha powder

1/2 cup coconut water

Directions:

Prepare the crust, and for this, place all its ingredients in a food processor and pulse for 3 to 5 minutes until the thick paste comes together.

Take a 6-inch springform pan, grease it with oil, place crust mixture in it and spread and press the mixture evenly in the bottom and along the sides, and freeze until required.

Prepare the filling and for this, place all its ingredients in a food processor, and pulse for 2 minutes until smooth.

Pour the filling into prepared pan, smooth the top, and freeze for 4 hours until set.

Cut pie into slices and then serve.

Nutrition:

Calories: 209 Cal

Fat: 18 g

Carbs: 10 g

Protein: 1 g

Fiber: 2 g

## Chocolate Peanut Butter Cake

Preparation time: 5 minutes

Cooking time: 0 minute

Servings: 8

Ingredients:

For the Base:

1 tablespoon ground flaxseeds

1/8 cup millet

3/4 cup peanuts

1/4 cup and 2 tablespoons shredded coconut unsweetened

1 teaspoon hemp oil

1/2 cup flake oats

For the Date Layer:

1 tablespoon ground flaxseed

1 cup dates

1 tablespoon hemp hearts

2 tablespoons coconut

3 tablespoons cacao

For the Chocolate Layer:

3/4 cup coconut flour

2 tablespoons and 2 teaspoons cacao

1 tablespoon maple syrup

8 tablespoons warm water

2 tablespoons coconut oil

1/2 cup coconut milk

2 tablespoons ground flaxseed

For the Chocolate Topping:

7 ounces coconut cream

2 1/2 tablespoons cacao

1 teaspoon agave

For Assembly:

1/2 cup almond butter

Directions:

Prepare the crust, and for this, place all its ingredients in a food processor and pulse for 3 to 5 minutes until the thick paste comes together.

Take a loaf tin, grease it with oil, place crust mixture in it and spread and press the mixture evenly in the bottom and along the sides, and freeze until required.

Prepare the date layer, and for this, place all its ingredients in a food processor and pulse for 2 minutes until smooth.

Prepare the chocolate layer, and for this, place flour and flax in a bowl and stir until combined.

Take a saucepan, add remaining ingredients, stir until mixed and Cooking Time: for 5 minutes until melted and smooth.

Add it into the flour mixture, stir until dough comes together, and set aside.

Prepare the chocolate topping, place all its ingredients in a food processor and pulse for 3 to 5 minutes until smooth.

Press date layer into the base layer, refrigerate for 1 hour, then press chocolate layer on its top, finish with chocolate topping, refrigerate for 3 hours and serve.

Nutrition:

Calories: 390 Cal

Fat: 24.3 g

Carbs: 35 g

Protein: 10.3 g

Fiber: 2 g

## Chocolate Raspberry Brownies

Preparation time: 4 hours

Cooking time: 0 minute

Servings: 4

Ingredients:

For the Chocolate Brownie Base:

12 Medjool Dates, pitted

3/4 cup oat flour

3/4 cup almond meal

3 tablespoons cacao

1 teaspoon vanilla extract, unsweetened

1/8 teaspoon sea salt

3 tablespoons water

1/2 cup pecans, chopped

For the Raspberry Cheesecake:

3/4 cup cashews, soaked, drained

6 tablespoons agave nectar

1/2 cup raspberries

1 teaspoon vanilla extract, unsweetened

1 lemon, juiced

6 tablespoons liquid coconut oil

For the Chocolate Coating:

2 1/2 tablespoons cacao powder

3 3/4 tablespoons coconut Oil

2 tablespoons maple syrup

1/8 teaspoon sea salt

Directions:

Prepare the crust, and for this, place all its ingredients in a food processor and pulse for 3 to 5 minutes until the thick paste comes together.

Take a 6-inch springform pan, grease it with oil, place crust mixture in it and spread and press the mixture evenly in the bottom and along the sides, and freeze until required.

Prepare the cheesecake topping, and for this, place all its ingredients in a food processor and pulse for 2 minutes until smooth.

Pour the filling into prepared pan, smooth the top, and freeze for 8 hours until solid.

Prepare the chocolate coating and for this, whisk together all its ingredients until smooth, drizzle on top of the cake and then serve.

Nutrition:

Calories: 371 Cal

Fat: 42.4 g

Carbs: 42 g

Protein: 5.5 g

Fiber: 2 g

**Brownie Batter**

Preparation time: 5 minutes

Cooking time: 0 minute

Servings: 4

Ingredients:

4 Medjool dates, pitted, soaked in warm water

1.5 ounces chocolate, unsweetened, melted

2 tablespoons maple syrup

4 tablespoons tahini

½ teaspoon vanilla extract, unsweetened

1 tablespoon cocoa powder, unsweetened

1/8 teaspoon sea salt

1/8 teaspoon espresso powder

2 to 4 tablespoons almond milk, unsweetened

Directions:

Place all the ingredients in a food processor and process for 2 minutes until combined.

Set aside until required.

Nutrition:

Calories: 44 Cal

Fat: 1 g

Carbs: 6 g

Protein: 2 g

Fiber: 0 g

## Strawberry Mousse

Preparation time: 5 minutes

Cooking time: 15 minutes

Servings: 4

Ingredients:

8 ounces coconut milk, unsweetened

2 tablespoons honey

5 strawberries

Directions:

Place berries in a blender and pulse until the smooth mixture comes together.

Place milk in a bowl, whisk until whipped, and then add remaining ingredients and stir until combined.

Refrigerate the mousse for 10 minutes and then serve.

Nutrition:

Calories: 145 Cal

Fat: 23 g

Carbs: 15 g

Protein: 5 g

Fiber: 1 g

**Blueberry Mousse**

Preparation time: 20 minutes

Cooking time: 0 minute

Servings: 2

Ingredients:

1 cup wild blueberries

1 cup cashews, soaked for 10 minutes, drained

1/2 teaspoon berry powder

2 tablespoons coconut oil, melted

1 tablespoon lemon juice

1 teaspoon vanilla extract, unsweetened

1/4 cup hot water

Directions:

Place all the ingredients in a food processor and process for 2 minutes until smooth.

Set aside until required.

Nutrition:

Calories: 433 Cal

Fat: 32.3 g

Carbs: 44 g

Protein: 5.1 g

Fiber: 0 g

# The Plant Based Soups and Salads Recipes

**Brussels Sprout Salad**

Servings: 4

Preparation time: 30 minutes

Cooking Time: 20 minutes

Ingredients:

For Salad

1 pound fresh medium Brussels sprouts, trimmed and vertically halved

4 tablespoons almond flour

3 teaspoons olive oil

2 apples, peeled and chopped

4 cups lettuce, torn

Salt and black pepper, to taste

1 red onion, sliced

For Dressing

2 tablespoons fresh lemon juice

2 tablespoons extra-virgin olive oil

1 tablespoon apple cider vinegar

1 tablespoon honey

Salt and black pepper, to taste

1 teaspoon Dijon mustard

Method:

Preheat the oven to 360 degrees F and grease a large baking sheet.

For Brussels sprout: Mix Brussels sprout, oil, salt, and black pepper in a bowl and toss to coat well.

Arrange the Brussels sprouts onto the baking sheet and transfer into the oven.

Bake for about 20 minutes, flipping once halfway through.

Remove from the oven and dish out the Brussel sprouts onto a plate.

Mix together the Brussel sprouts, apples, onion, and lettuce in a serving bowl.

For dressing: Combine all the ingredients in a bowl and beat until well combined.

Pour the dressing into the Brussels sprouts and stir well to serve.

Nutrition Information per Serving:

Calories:217

Fat: 7.7g

Carbohydrates: 36g

Fibers: 8.7g

Sugar:20.3g

Protein: 6.4g

Sodium: 52mg

## Lentil Soup

Servings:3

Preparation time: 15 minutes

Cooking Time: 40 minutes

Ingredients:

2 leeks, chopped

¼ cup brown lentils

½ bunch fresh kale, trimmed and chopped

Salt and black pepper, to taste

1 tablespoon vegetable oil

1 (14-ounce) can whole tomatoes, drained

3 cups vegetable broth

1 sweet potato, peeled and cubed

½ tablespoon fresh thyme, chopped

Method:

Heat the oil over medium heat in a large soup pan and add the leeks.

Sauté for about 4 minutes and add the tomatoes.

Cooking Time: for about 6 minutes, stirring constantly and stir in the broth.

Bring to a boil and add the sweet potato, lentils, thyme and kale.

Bring to a boil again and reduce the heat to low.

Cover the pan and allow to simmer for about 30 minutes.

Season with salt and black pepper and dish out to serve hot.

Nutrition Information per Serving:

Calories: 189

Net Carbs: 19g

Fat: 6.5g

Carbohydrates: 25.5g

Fiber: 4.5g Sugar: 9.3g

Protein: 8.6g

Sodium: 842mg

**Egg-Plant Salad**

Servings:                                                                                    2

Preparation time: 30 minutes

Cooking Time: 25 minutes

Ingredients:

For Salad

2 tablespoons canola oil

1 eggplant, cut crosswise into ½-inch-thick slices

Salt and black pepper, to taste

1 teaspoon fresh lemon juice

1 avocado, peeled, pitted and chopped

For Dressing

1 tablespoon extra-virgin olive oil

1 tablespoon red wine vinegar

1 tablespoon honey

1 teaspoon fresh lemon zest, grated

1 tablespoon fresh oregano leaves, chopped

Salt and black pepper, to taste

1 teaspoon Dijon mustard

Method:

Preheat the oven to 360 degrees F and grease a baking pan lightly.

For Salad: Put the eggplant, oil, salt, and black pepper in a bowl and toss to coat well.

Arrange the eggplants pieces into the baking pan in a single layer and transfer into the oven.

Bake for about 25 minutes and remove from the oven.

Mix the avocado and lemon juice in a bowl and add the eggplants pieces.

For Dressing: Put all the ingredients in a bowl and beat until well combined.

Pour the dressing onto the eggplants mixture and combine well to serve.

Nutrition Information per Serving:

Calories: 489

Net Carbs: 14.7

Dietary Fibers: 16g

Fat: 41.4g

Carbohydrates: 32.7g

Sugar: 16.2g

Protein: 4.6g

Sodium: 41mg

Cabbage Carrot Salad

Servings: 4

Preparation time: 15 minutes

Ingredients:

2 cups purple cabbage, shredded

2 cups green cabbage, shredded

2 cups carrot, peeled and chopped

2 large scallions, chopped

¼ cup fresh cilantro leaves, chopped

1 jalapeño pepper, seeded and minced

2 tablespoons fresh lemon juice

2 tablespoons extra-virgin olive oil

Salt and freshly ground black pepper, to taste

2 tablespoons walnuts, chopped

1 teaspoon fresh lemon zest, grated finely

Method:

In a large serving bowl, add all the ingredients except lemon zest and toss to coat well.

Serve with the garnishing of walnuts and lemon zest.

Nutrition Information per Serving:

Calories: 123Net Carbs: 6.3g

Fat: 9.5gSugar: 4.5g

Fiber: 3g Carbohydrates: 9.3g

Protein: 2.2gSodium: 48mg


**Chickpeas Soup**

Servings: 6

Preparation time: 15 minutes

Cooking Time: 55 minutes

Ingredients:

3 tablespoons vegetable oil

1 large onion, chopped

8 garlic cloves, minced

1 teaspoon ground cumin

1 teaspoon ground cinnamon

1 teaspoon sweet paprika

1/8 teaspoon cayenne pepper

3 (15-ounce) cans chickpeas, rinsed and drained

1 (14½-ounce) can diced tomatoes with liquid

1 teaspoon sugar

Salt and black pepper, to taste

4½ cups vegetable broth

1 (5-ounce) package fresh baby spinach

2 tablespoons fresh lemon juice

Method:

Heat oil in a large soup pan over medium heat and add onion.

Sauté for about 5 minutes and add garlic and spices.

Sauté for about 1 minute and stir in the tomatoes, chickpeas, sugar, broth, salt and black pepper.

Bring to a boil and lower the heat.

Allow to simmer for about 45 minutes and remove from the heat.

Dish out half of the chickpeas into a bowl and blend them with a potato masher.

Return the mashed chickpeas into the pan with remaining soup and stir well.

Place the pan over medium heat and add the spinach.

Allow to simmer for about 4 minutes and sprinkle with salt and black pepper.

Remove from the heat and drizzle with lemon juice to serve hot.


Nutrition Information per Serving:

Calories: 894

Net Carbs: 95.5g

Fat: 21g

Carbohydrates: 136.2g

Fiber: 38.7g

Sugar: 25.7g

Protein: 46.2g

Sodium: 646mg

**Fruity Spinach Salad**

Servings: 8

Preparation time: 15 minutes

Ingredients:

3 cups fresh mango, peeled, pitted and cubed

3 cups fresh pineapple, peeled and chopped

12 cups fresh baby spinach

½ cup fresh mint leaves, chopped

4 tablespoons fresh orange juice

½ cup dried cranberries

Salt, to taste

Method:

Put all the ingredients in a large serving bowl and toss to coat well.

Cover the bowl and refrigerate for about 1 hour before serving.

Nutrition Information per Serving:

Calories: 88

Net Carbs: 15.4g

Fat: 0.6g

Carbohydrates: 20.9g

Fiber: 3.5g

Sugar: 15.6g

Protein: 2.4g

Sodium: 58mg

## Mixed Beans Soup

Servings: 12

Preparation time: 15 minutes

Cooking Time: 30 minutes

Ingredients:

1 onion, chopped

3 celery stalks, chopped

¼ cup vegetable oil

2 large potatoes, scrubbed and cubed

3 carrots, peeled and chopped

3 garlic cloves, minced

1 (4-ounce) can green chilies

1 tablespoon ground cumin

2 (16-ounce) cans great Northern beans, rinsed and drained

1 (15-ounce) can black beans, rinsed and drained

4 cups vegetable broth

1 cup red wine

2 teaspoons dried thyme, crushed

2 jalapeño peppers, chopped

2 (15-ounce) cans red kidney beans, rinsed and drained

15-ounce tomato-vegetable juice cocktail

2 tablespoons brown sugar

Method:

Heat vegetable oil in a large soup pan over medium heat and add the onion, potatoes, carrot and celery.

Sauté for about 4 minutes and add the garlic, green chilies, thyme, cumin and jalapeño peppers.

Sauté for about 1 minute and stir in the beans, juice cocktail, broth and brown sugar.

Bring to a boil and cook, covered for about 25 minutes.

Stir in the red wine and dish out to serve hot.

Nutrition Information per Serving:

Calories: 786

Net Carbs: 99.3g

Fat: 7.9g

Carbohydrates: 136.1g

Fiber: 36.8g Sugar: 12.9g

Protein: 44.5gS

odium: 461mg

**Potato Salad**

Servings: 6

Preparation time: 35 minutes

Cooking Time: 40 minutes

Ingredients:

1 tablespoon olive oil

4 Russet potatoes

Salt, to taste

3 hard-boiled eggs, peeled and chopped

½ cup red onion, chopped

¼ teaspoon celery salt

¼ cup mayonnaise

1 cup celery, chopped

1 tablespoon prepared mustard

¼ teaspoon garlic salt

Method:

Preheat the oven to 360 degrees F and grease a large baking sheet.

Prick the potatoes with a fork, drizzle with oil and season with salt.

Arrange the potatoes on the baking sheet and transfer

into the oven.

Bake for about 40 minutes and dish out in a bowl.

Chop the potatoes after cooling and stir in the remaining ingredients.

Mix well and refrigerate to chill before serving.

Nutrition Information per Serving:

Calories: 196

Net Carbs: 20.5g

Fat: 8.1g

Carbohydrates: 26.5g

Fiber: 4g

Sugar: 3.1g

Protein: 5.6g

Sodium: 18mg

**Beans and Parsley Soup**

Servings: 4

Preparation time: 15 minutes

Cooking Time: 40 minutes

Ingredients:

2 tablespoons coconut oil

2 tablespoons fresh rosemary, chopped

2 cups canned white beans, rinsed and drained

2 garlic cloves, minced

¼ cup fresh parsley leaves, chopped

1 white onion, chopped

2 celery stalks, chopped

1 large carrot, peeled and chopped

4 cups vegetable broth

2 tablespoons fresh lemon juice

4 cups fresh tomatoes, chopped finely

1 cup pearl barley

Method:

Heat coconut oil over medium heat in a large soup pan and add onion, celery and carrot.

Sauté for about 5 minutes and add garlic and rosemary.

Sauté for about 1 minute and stir in the tomatoes.

Cooking Time: for 4 minutes, stirring continuously and add the broth and barley.

Bring to a boil and reduce the heat to low.

Cover the lid and allow to simmer for about 25 minutes.

Stir in the lemon juice and beans and simmer for about 5 minutes.

Remove from the heat and garnish with parsley to serve.

Nutrition Information per Serving:

Calories: 672

Net Carbs: 84.8g

Fat: 10.4g

Carbohydrates: 114.2g

Fiber: 27.4g Sugar: 10.3g

Protein: 35.8gSodium: 818mg


**Cauliflower Salad**

Servings: 4

Preparation time: 25 minutes

Cooking Time: 20 minutes

Ingredients:

For Salad

1 cup boiling water

¼ cup golden raisins

¼ cup olive oil

1 head cauliflower, cut into small florets

Salt, to taste

2 tablespoons fresh mint leaves

1 tablespoon curry powder

¼ cup pecans, toasted and chopped

For Dressing

1 cup mayonnaise

1 tablespoon fresh lemon juice

2 tablespoons sugar

Method:

Preheat the oven to 390 degrees F and grease a large baking sheet.

Arrange the cauliflower florets on the baking sheet in a single layer and transfer into the oven.

Bake for about 20 minutes and dish out in a bowl.

Meanwhile, soak the raisins in boiling water in a bowl and keep aside.

For Dressing: Mix all the ingredients in a bowl until well combined.

Mix the cauliflower, raisins and pecans in another bowl and pour in the dressing.

Stir well to combine and garnish with mint.

Refrigerate to chill before serving.

Nutrition Information per Serving:

Calories: 417

Net Carbs: 27.3g

Fat: 33.2g

Carbohydrates: 32.1g

Fiber: 2.8g Sugar: 16.9g

Protein: 2.5g

Sodium: 482mg

## Lentil and Barley Soup

Servings:4

Preparation time: 20 minutes

Cooking Time: 50 minutes

Ingredients:

1 carrot, peeled and chopped

½ large onion, chopped

1 celery stalk, chopped

1 garlic clove, minced

½ cup barley

4 cups vegetable broth

½ teaspoon ground coriander

½ teaspoon cayenne pepper

2 cups fresh spinach, torn

1 teaspoon ground cumin

½ cup red lentils

1 tablespoon olive oil

Salt and black pepper, to taste

½ (14-ounce) can diced tomatoes with liquid

Method:

Heat olive oil in a large pan over medium heat and add the carrots, onion and celery.

Sauté for about 5 minutes and add garlic and spices.

Sauté for about 1 minute and stir in the lentils, barley, tomatoes and broth.

Bring to a boil and lower the heat.

Cover the lid and allow to simmer for about 40 minutes.

Stir in the spinach, salt and black pepper and simmer for about 4 minutes.

Remove from the heat and dish out to serve hot.

Nutrition Information per Serving:

Calories: 278

Net Carbs: 25.5g

Fat: 6.2g

Carbohydrates: 41.6g

Fiber: 14.1g S

Sugar: 6.3g

Protein: 16g

Sodium: 801mg

## Zucchini Salad

Servings: 4

Preparation time: 45minutes

Ingredients:

1 teaspoon garlic powder

1 pound zucchini, cut into rounds

2 tablespoons olive oil

5 cups fresh spinach, chopped

2 tablespoons fresh lemon juice

Salt and black pepper, as required

¼ cup feta cheese, crumbled

Method:

Preheat the oven to 400 degrees F and grease a large baking sheet.

Mix zucchini, oil, garlic powder, salt, and black pepper in a bowl.

Arrange the zucchini slices on the baking sheet in a single layer and transfer into the oven.

Bake for about 30 minutes and dish out in a serving plate.

Add spinach, feta cheese, lemon juice, a little bit of salt, and black pepper to zucchini slices and toss well to serve.

Nutrition Information per Serving:

Calories: 116

Net Carbs: 5.1gFat: 9.4g

Carbohydrates: 6.2g

Fiber: 0.9g Sugar: 2.5g

Protein: 4gSodium: 186mg

## Beans and Pasta Soup

Servings: 6

Preparation time: 15 minutes

Cooking Time: 15 minutes

Ingredients:

2 teaspoons vegetable oil

4 garlic cloves, minced

1 teaspoon dried rosemary, crushed

1/8 teaspoon paprika

2 (15-ounce) cans navy beans, rinsed and drained

1 cup orzo pasta

1 large leek, chopped

¼ teaspoon red pepper flakes, crushed

4 cups vegetable broth

1 (28-ounce) can diced tomatoes

Salt and black pepper, to taste

Method:

Heat vegetable oil in a large soup pan over medium heat and add the leeks, garlic, rosemary and spices.

Sauté for about 3 minutes and stir in the broth.

Bring to a boil and boil for about 2 minutes.

Add beans, tomatoes and pasta and Cooking Time: for about 10 minutes.

Season with salt and black pepper and dish out to serve hot.

Nutrition Information per Serving:

Calories: 615Net Carbs: 69.9g

Fat: 5.4gCarbohydrates: 106.5g

Fiber: 36.6g Sugar: 10.1g

Protein: 38.8gSodium: 531mg

## Tomato & Mozzarella Salad

Yield: 6 servings

Preparation time: 15 minutes

Ingredients:

1½ pounds mozzarella cheese, cubed

4 cups cherry tomatoes, halved

¼ cup fresh basil leaves, chopped

¼ cup olive oil

1 teaspoon fresh oregano, minced

4 drops liquid stevia

2 tablespoons fresh lemon juice

1 teaspoon fresh parsley, minced

Salt and black pepper, to taste

Method:

Mix tomatoes, mozzarella cheese and basil a large salad bowl.

For Dressing: Mix the remaining ingredients in a small bowl and beat until well combined.

Pour the dressing over salad and mix well to serve immediately.

Nutrition Information per Serving:

Calories: 116Net Carbs: 1.6g

Fat: 10gCarbohydrates: 5.2g

Fiber: 1.6gSugar: 3.3g

Protein: 3.2gSodium: 50mg


## Vegetable Tortilla Soup

Servings: 4

Preparation time: 5 minutes

Cooking Time: 30 minutes

Ingredients:

2 tablespoons olive tomato paste

1/2 can, roasted tomatoes

1 quart vegetable broth

1/2 teaspoon kosher salt

Freshly ground black pepper

9 ounces good-quality fresh tortellini

1 handful basil leaves

black pepper, ground

2 celery stalks, chopped

1 onion, diced

2 carrots, peeled

2 garlic cloves, minced

2 tablespoons olive oil

1 teaspoon paprika

Method:

Take a frying pan, add oil to it.

Turn on the stove; sauté the onion and garlic with the tomato paste and paprika over medium-low heat for 5 minutes.

Add carrots and celery to it and sauté again for 5 more minutes.

Take another pan, add tomatoes, vegetable broth, kosher salt, and black pepper to it. Let it boil and then simmer for 15 minutes.

Cooking Time: tortellini according to the instruction.

Mix all the contents together.

Stir in basil leaves.

Drizzle oil on it.

Serve hot!

Nutrition Information per Serving:

Calories: 324

Net Carbs: 32.9

Fat: 11.8g

Carbohydrates: 40.2g

Sugar: 5.3g

Protein: 12.2g


**Creamy Vegan Broccoli Soup**

Servings: 8

time: 15 minutes

Ingredients:

¼ cup olive oil

4 cups vegetable broth

2 cups non-dairy milk

¾ cup coconut milk

¼ cup nutritional yeast flakes

1 teaspoon lemon juice

5 cups broccoli, chopped

2/3 cup carrots, chopped

2/3 cup celery, chopped

2/3 cups onion, chopped

2 cloves garlic, minced

6 tablespoon flour

½ teaspoon salt

Black pepper, to taste

Method:

Heat olive oil over medium heat and sauté broccoli, carrot, celery, onion, and garlic in it for 5 minutes

Sprinkle flour over the vegetables and Cooking Time: for 2 minutes.

Add vegetable broth, non-dairy milk, coconut milk and

nutritional yeast, stir continuously.

Simmer soup for 15 minutes and let the vegetables to soften.

Blend the soup for 2 minutes, and add white vinegar.

Add salt and pepper finally.

Serve hot!

Nutrition Information per Serving:

Calories: 219

Net Carbs: 10.9g

Fat: 13.8g

Carbohydrates: 17.1g

Fiber: 4.2g

Sugar: 5.1g

Protein: 9.5g

Sodium: 599mg

**No-Cooking Time: Chickpea Salad**

Servings: 6

Preparation time: 10 minutes

Cooking Time: 0 minutes

Ingredients:

2 large tomatoes, chopped

2 tablespoons olive oil

2 tablespoons harissa

1 can chickpeas, drained

1 lemon, juiced

1 bunch coriander, chopped

1 bunch parsley, chopped

1 red onion, sliced

Method:

Mash chickpeas a little so that they do not remain harder.

Mix all the vegetables together.

Add lemon juice to it.

Serve and enjoy!

Nutrition Information per Serving:

Calories: 200

Net Carbs: 18.2

Fat: 7.7g

Carbohydrates: 27.5g

Sugar: 7.6g

Protein: 7.7g

Sodium: 74g

Fibers: 7.3


**Carrot, Pea, and Mint Salad**

Servings: 4

Preparation time: 15 minutes

Ingredients:

2 teaspoons agave nectar

2 tablespoons lemon juice, freshly squeezed

6 tablespoons extra virgin olive oil

½ teaspoon salt

¼ teaspoon freshly ground black pepper

2 tablespoons fresh mint, chopped

4 medium carrots, peeled and thinly sliced

2 cups frozen peas, defrosted and boiled

Method:

Whisk together agave nectar, olive oil, lemon juice, mint, salt and black pepper in a large bowl.

Toss to coat well and dish out in a serving platter to serve.

Nutrition Information per Serving:

Calories: 301

Net Carbs: 17.2g

Fat: 21.3g

Carbohydrates: 25.9g

Fiber: 6.7g

Sugar: 14.4g

Protein: 4.8g

Sodium: 393mg

# *Tips and Tricks*

Before we send you on your way to your new healthy lifestyle, there are a few important tips and tricks for you to learn and keep up your sleeve. In the beginning, it always seems easy to begin a new diet. You have this new found motivation and energy to change your life. But, what happens when that energy burns out in a few weeks? By knowing some tips and tricks about the plant-based diet, these will keep you going when times get rough!

Getting Started on a Plant-based Diet

1.    Find Your Motivation

Truly, I cannot express the importance of this enough! If you are here in this book, there was probably something drastic that made you want to make a major change. This reason is your why and what you should set your goals around. Whether you are looking for mental clarity, more energy, or helping a disease, always try to remember why you are starting this lifestyle in the first place. For bonus points, write down your why on a sheet of paper so that you can look at it when you need added motivation.

2.    Remember to Eat

As mentioned earlier, a plant-based diet is very filling when you are consuming whole foods. It will be important that you remember to eat more than you are used to. Luckily on a plant-based diet, you can say goodbye to counting calories. Now, you can fill up on salad, fruit, quinoa, beans, and even baked potatoes to your heart's content! The whole point of this diet is to live off the good food, and over time, the body adjusts to the volume of food. After a while, you will learn to rely on your satiety cues and natural hunger.

3.    Prepare Food

As you start a plant-based diet, I encourage you to take a stroll through your kitchen. In the beginning, you will begin to recognize the foods that may not be as beneficial to you as a whole food. I suggest you toss these foods or give them away, so you keep yourself out of temptations reach. Instead, fill your fridge and pantry with healthy foods such as beans, rice, and potatoes! This way when you get cravings for unhealthy foods, there won't be any in your house!

4.    Take it Gentle

Switching over to a plant-based diet does not need to happen overnight! Instead, I suggest taking a gentler approach and slowly switch your diet to become more plant-based. If you make sudden changes, you could potentially feel restricted and ultimately cheat yourself out of your amazing diet. An example would be to use avocado instead of butter! While it is a change, it will take some time to get used to. As you increase the healthy plant-based ingredients in your life, you will slowly eliminate the bad stuff.

5.    One Meal at a Time

There are no rules saying that being plant-based needs to be a now or never type of deal. Instead, try switching one meal at a time to be more plant-based. One of the easier meals, I have found, is breakfast! Instead of your normal milk and cereal, give oatmeal with your favorite fruit a try! There is also delicious avocado toast or breakfast potatoes! I highly suggest trying some of the recipes provided in this book to help you get started! Slowly, you can switch all of your meals to being plant-based, and soon it won't even be a second thought.

6.    Find Good People

I mentioned earlier that many people close to you will doubt your lifestyle choice, but there are also many likeminded people out there in the world that are going through the same changes as you. Typically, it is easier to go through changes when you have company to share your struggles and successes with. It is a fantastic idea to form a support group so you can reach out for help and inspire others. I suggest checking out internet forums or even Facebook groups for you to connect with. Just remember that you are never alone on this journey!

7.    Keep it Fun

Switching to a plant-based diet is not meant to be a form of torture. I hope that eventually, you learn to enjoy your food choices and perhaps even look forward to it. Luckily with modern technology, you have recipes at your fingertips. There are always new foods to try and recipes to give a shot. A good way to keep your diet fun is to have an adventurous side. The next time you visit the grocery store, I challenge you to choose out a fruit or vegetable that you have never heard of before. When you have made your selection, use the internet to find ideas on how to Cooking Time: this item. You may be surprised at what you learn about food and about yourself!

8.    Commit

As you begin the plant-based diet, the best thing you can do is make the commitment to yourself. There are a number of reasons people begin the plant-based diet. Why are you here? Why do you feel a plant-based diet can change your life? At the end of the day, it does not matter what anyone else thinks. If you want to make this commitment to yourself, you make this commitment! It is time to take your health into your own hands. You are the only one who can make health decisions for yourself, make sure those decisions are the best ones possible. You owe yourself that much.

Plant-based on a Budget

One major excuse individuals use not to eat healthily is that they feel eating healthy can be too expensive. The trick here is to make smart choices. There are plenty of ways to strip the diet down to the basics; whole foods can actually be easily affordable for just about anyone! All you need is some knowledge about whole foods, and you will be able to fit all of your nutrients into your budget with ease!

1.    Stay Home!

This seems like a given but eating at home instead of going out to a restaurant can save you a lot of money whether you follow a plant-based diet or not! Instead of dining out several times a week, eat out for an occasional treat! If you are constantly on the move and rely on fast food, begin to prepare snacks in advance. This way, you will have full control over your meals and what goes into them. Also, by staying home, this will give you a fantastic chance to work on those cooking skills!

2.    Choose Whole Foods

While this may seem like a given, whole foods are going to be some of the cheapest staples you can buy! Luckily, the whole foods are going to offer the most essential nutrients as well! Some of the more popular, budget-friendly foods include brown rice, oats, potatoes, carrots, leafy greens, frozen vegetables, apples, oranges, other fruits in season, and all of the beans and lentils!

3.    Think Big

Not literally, but when you buy food in bulk, you can get much more bang for your buck! When you are at the grocery store, look for the big packages or family packs. Typically, these will provide better value compared to smaller bags or containers. In this case, you will want to pay special attention to the unit price located on the price tag; this number will tell you the cost per pound. By following this rule, you can choose the cheapest option.

4.    Keep it Simple, Stupid

If you are just starting the plant-based diet, there is no reason to get crazy and wild in the kitchen! Just because you are switching your diet, this does not mean that you need to become a crazy, skilled chef. Keeping your meals simple does not mean that they are going to be boring. As you can tell from the recipes earlier in this book, recipes can be easy and delicious at the same time. Often times when you use too many ingredients, this makes it tough on the pallet and your digestion tract. Do yourself a favor and start small. As you get better with this lifestyle, that is when you can experiment a bit more with your meals.

5.    Buy in Season

This is vital when it comes to shopping for a plant-based diet on a budget. The good news is that food that is grown in season is cheaper and tastes much better. In the winter, keep an eye out for citrus fruits and root vegetables. In the summer, you can keep your eyes out for nectarines and watermelon. Do yourself a favor and visit your local farmers market to get the freshest produce possible. You may be surprised to learn the wide variety of food that is made available to you!

6.      Frozen

Lastly, frozen fruits and vegetables. These items are typically cheaper and can be very convenient. Frozen fruits and vegetables are typically picked once they are ripe and then frozen right away; this meaning that the foods will maintain their nutrition. This is a fantastic idea, especially in the winter when fresh produce may be limited on variety and quality. Just remember to read the label of ingredients so you can avoid any added butter, sauce, or seasoning.

# *Conclusion*

The plant-based diet in reality isn't a tough one to practice. To me, it comes across as the easiest way to diet for food prep and digestion. Plant foods Cooking Time: the fastest and are easy to grasp for beginner cooks.

While there might be arguments as to the plant-based diet being a vegan, vegetarian, plant to animal-based, or a partially processed foods diet, the plant-based diet stands as a unique one by itself. It combines and eliminates aspects of all four of these ways of eating to create a wholesome approach that servings: the body better.

In my opinion, it is one that eliminates the presence of animal and processed foods in meals but incorporates plant-foods to the best possible. Now, will you question if these dishes will be tasty? I can guarantee with full backing that the WFPB offers some of the most delicious foods that there are. Think of fresh crunchy salads with super tasty dressings, scrumptious soups that incorporate plant creams, nuts, and seeds for mouthwatering sips, and the list is endless.

While I have found the plant-based diet to be more nutritious than regular diets, it offers tremendous benefits that servings: as a proof for longevity too. Counting the benefits, it facilitates weight loss, reduces the risk of heart diseases, cancers, and cognitive decline. In addition, for the high amounts of nutrients present in plant foods, they result in the right nutritional balance within the body.

Beginning the whole foods plant-based diet is as easy as tucking away all the animal and processed foods that you previously enjoyed and replacing them with plant-based options.

It is a fun world with these recipes! I am happy that I can share them with you and look forward to the exciting foods that you make.  Don't forget to prep your mind, self, and kitchen in ways that will make it a fun journey for you. Consider the lifestyle as an adventure and take it one step at a time. Also, create a small community of similar dieters that will encourage you on this path. Meanwhile, own your kitchen and make it a paradise for your plant-based food preps. I can guarantee that you will enjoy walking into your kitchen often and you will magically create foods that will leave you wanting more.

This Plant-Based Cookbook for Beginners will be your companion for many days to come! Now, it is time for me to say a goodbye but not quite a goodbye. I am heading out to create my next exciting cookbook on a topic that I know will excite you as much as this. You should look out for it!

# The Plant Based Diet Meal Plan

*The New Vegetable Diet Cookbook with Vegan, Fat Free Vegan and Low Carbs Recipes to Burn Fat, Stimulate Weight Loss and Energy Reset*

## SEBI ALAN GUNTRY

# Tables of Contents

# *Introduction*

Plant-based weight control plans offer all the essential protein, fats, carbohydrates, nutrients, and minerals for ideal wellbeing, and are regularly higher in fiber and phytonutrients. Notwithstanding, a few vegans may need to include an enhancement (explicitly nutrient B12) to guarantee they get every one of the nutrients required.

There is no reasonable meaning of what comprises an entire nourishment, plant-based eating regimen (WFPB diet). The WFPB diet isn't really a set eating regimen — it's to a greater degree a way of life. This is on the grounds that plant-based eating regimens can shift enormously relying upon the degree to which an individual incorporates creature items in their eating regimen.

Regardless, the essential standards of an entire nourishments, plant-based diet are as per the following:

Emphasizes entire, negligibly handled nourishments.

Limits or stays away from creature items.

Excludes refined nourishments, as included sugars, white flour and handled oils.

Pays extraordinary consideration regarding nourishment quality, with numerous advocates of the WFPB diet advancing privately sourced, natural nourishment at whatever point conceivable.

Hence, this eating regimen is regularly mistaken for vegan or vegetarian eats less. However, albeit comparable here and there, these weight control plans are not the equivalent.

For all the vegetarians and plant lovers, there is a plant-based diet plan available that helps them to get better and in good shape. The new form of vegetarian diet helps the people to look great, stay active and be healthy. It is an all plant and no meat diet that is easy to digest, fresh and gives numerous benefits as well.

Normally, people consider that plants come with limited options but in reality, it is very different. For a hardcore plant-based food plan there are numerous options available for a person. These ground growing food items have numerous nutrition, vitamins and other resources in them that are not measurable. If a person is good enough to prepare a list of ultimate food options and get the right guide for the plant-based diet, they will get maximum benefit.

Here in this book, you can find everything you need to know about the plant-based diet. From its basics to the ultimate diet plans and recipes there is everything available of your interest. It is a composite and complete resource for you that help you to follow the diet plan in all healthy manners and take full advantage of it. All you need is to go through these resources and manage everything as per your own preferences.

People have over time managed to interpret plant-based meals to other products that are inclusive of meat in the diet. That remains a controversy as different cultures have different beliefs. The rise of processed foods over the years has brought deceases and other challenges in the food industry. This is the reason why a good number of individuals have decided to turn to plant-based meals as they believe it reduces the chances of diseases and well as it being cost-effective in one way or another. People will argue that there is no difference in a full meal diet and a plant-based meal, but science has proven that they are indeed different.

Plant-based meals are considered to be healthier as compared to other types of meals. Fast food is the order of the day as the human race has become so busy to even take a look on their health meaning that it is possible for a large population to have grown far away from healthy living. This book emphasizes the importance of a healthy lifestyle as well as gives instructions on how to change and start on the journey of healthy living by incorporating a plant-based meal in each and everyone's meal plans. By choosing a healthy lifestyle, a person will be able to be in control of their body fat content and also check their weight as this will be more beneficial to them in a healthy way and guarantee them a life that is less of strange diseases with lots of expenses on drugs and checkups.

# Chapter 1 The Plant-based Diet: How Can It Improve My Lifestyle?

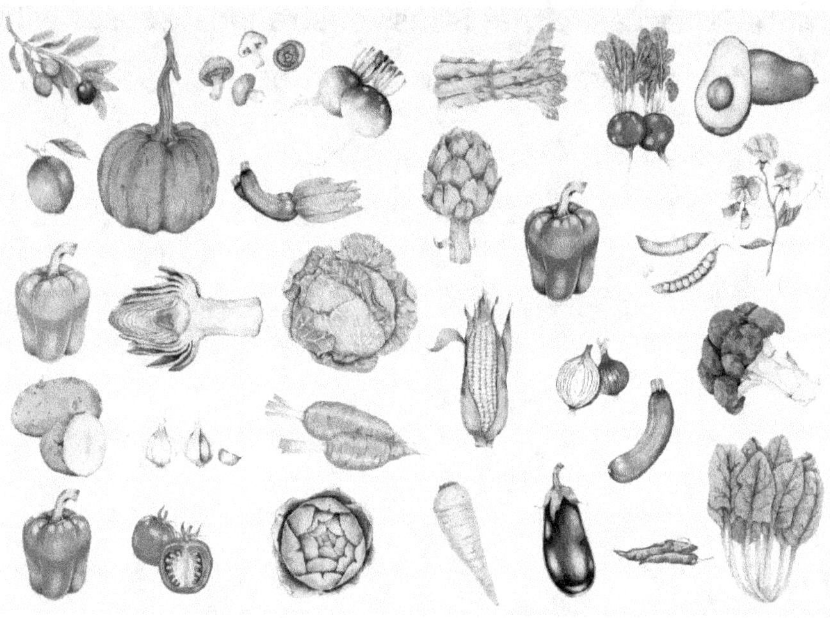

The plant-based diet is a style of eating that focuses entirely on food from plants. Foods in this category include fruits, nuts, seeds grains, legumes, vegetables, oils, and beans.

The plant-based diet is different from a vegan or vegetarian plan because a plant-based diet doesn't forbid eating animal products; it allows you to choose a more proportionate amount of plant-sourced food in your diet.

People understand and use the phrase plant-based diet in a variety of ways; a lot of people take the name literally. For most of those people, the plant-based diet is like a vegan diet where no animal products are involved. But the truth is that the person who is following a plant-based diet can consume chicken, meat, or fish occasionally. The main focus is on the whole and healthy food items rather than the processed items.

# Chapter 2 Why a Plant-Based Diet?

Why not? The health benefits associated with this diet make it one of the most highly recommended diet plans to follow.

The plant-based diet has very few restrictions, and it is not expensive to follow.

The meal plans are healthy, delicious, and good for your body.

The plant-based diet is high in fiber, water, and complex carbohydrates, which help the person to remain full for a longer period.

It is highly recommended for aged people, teenagers, nursing moms, and pregnant women.

A lot of research and evidence prove that it helps to lose weight effectively.

People who eat plant-based diets have low BMI, lower rates of heart disease, and lower cholesterol.

It is also effective in helping to prevent and manage diabetes.

## Starting a Diet and Weight Loss

Starting a plant-based diet is easy: you do not need to eliminate huge food categories, and you do not need to subscribe to any expensive online plan. You need to follow these simple steps to get started with the diet plan:

Add more fruits and vegetables to your diet.

Start the day with a bowl of salad or soup.

Always cook a meal in oils that are plant-based like canola, olive oil, and peanut oil.

If you feel, need to munch on something, choose nuts and seeds for snacking.

For breakfast, choose tea and coffee that is unsweetened and without animal milk.

The meal should be comprised of those food items that are organic, whole, and full of vitamins, minerals, and protein.

You may add limited sweet treats. It's better to satisfy the sweet craving with fruit-based desserts and drinks.

It is highly recommended to only have 5-10% of the calories in your meal be from meat.

Try to include grain and legumes.

Choose your breakfast wisely by adding bread made with buckwheat, barley, or wheat.

"Go green" is the tagline for a vegan diet plan, and it is the best choice possible for healthy foods.

## Advantages/benefits of Plant-Based Diet and Its Usefulness

Prevent hypertension

The addition of healthy green vegetables, fruits, and healthy unprocessed food items contribute toward low blood pressure. When a person switches to a plant-based diet, it automatically reduces the blood pressure and increases the potassium. The potassium helps in lowering hypertension and anxiety. The nuts, legume, and grains provide vitamin b6 that helps to lower the blood pressure.

Effective weight loss

Different research and study conduct that people following a plant-based diet tend to have a very low body mass index and have lower chances of getting obese. They also tend to have a very low rate of heart disease and diabetes. The plant-based diet plan is rich in fiber, protein, minerals, and calcium. All these nutrients make the body feel fuller for a longer period. It is one of the effective diets that treats obesity and reduces excess weight.

More energy and efficiency

The food groups that are part of the plant-based diet are rich in good fats and nutrients that provide instant energy to the body and cutting down the meat; you can reap a lot of health benefits.

Lower the rate of cancer and cardiovascular diseases.

The good fat and omega 3 rich food help lower the fat. The whole foods plant-based diet improves the chances of avoiding cancer as we cut on red meat, smoking, and alcohol, and we all know all these items are a link to increased heart diseases.

## Differences with Other Diets

Vegetarian

A plant-based diet is totally different from a vegetarian diet. The main difference is that vegetarians eat some animal products such as honey and milk while a plant-based diet is exclusively made of plant products only.

Vegan

There has often been some confusion as to whether the plant-based diet is just another word for veganism, or if they are a completely different concept with different rules, so let's go into that. There are many similarities between the two, but also some distinct differences. Are veganism and a plant-based diet the same thing? The short answer is no. The particular diet that is chosen and the label it is given depends on the individual, and the reason they have chosen to live this lifestyle. Many vegans choose to be so because they disagree with the slaughter and poor treatment of farm animals, and so they do not consume these foods. They also usually choose not to use leather or wear fur or any other animal products. Vegans do not eat any sort of meat, or product containing traces of meat. This includes any broths or ingredients such as gelatin. Vegans also do not eat any food products that contain ANY ingredient from an animal, including milk or honey. They do not eat any cheese, or yogurt, or margarine or butter, etc. Some slightly more hidden ingredients that contain animal products are whey and casein. These are all avoided. Vegans get most of their food from plant sources, but they are not strictly whole food plant based. They may not be as health conscious, and so many may choose to eat packaged and processed foods, yet stay away from those made of animals. This technically still falls within the parameter of their diet.

Plant-based folks eat a primarily plant derived diet- as close to nature as possible. But this does not mean that they are vegan, or even vegetarian. They may simply choose to eat mostly fruits, vegetables, nuts and legumes, etc. However, they may still choose to eat meat, and carefully choose meats that are antibiotics free, grass fed, and lived a free-range life. Many plant-based dieters believe that meat is still an integral part of a healthy diet, and so they just choose the best quality possible.

Whole food, plant-based diets usually take the qualities of both diets and even go a step further. Keeping foods whole refers to leaving them in their most natural state. So, vegetables and fruit are eaten as they are fresh, frozen or dried without preservatives or added flavor. Nuts are natural, without salt or sugar; grains are not refined or enriched or bleached. Most foods are prepared at home, or in a restaurant where the chefs share the same standards, as to not degrade any of the ingredients or take away any of their nutritional value. Many processed foods use what is known as plant fragments, rather than whole plants. They are reduced, or extracted or otherwise processed in some way.

Whatever the specifics of the diet someone chooses, if they tell you that they are vegan or plant based, you should assume that they do not consume any animal products at all, unless they mention it otherwise. This can help you to avoid accidentally serving them something that they will not be willing or able to eat. And feel free to ask someone about their diet, if you are curious. But make sure that they are willing to talk about it, and also that you listen with an open mind-not looking to judge or challenge their decision to adopt that particular diet.

Pescatarian

The pescatarians adhere to a diet with seafood as the sole meat source. It is clearly different from a plant-based diet because it incorporates seafood and eggs dairy products, which are not part of the plant-based diet. Pescatarians cannot eat other meat apart from seafood.

Flexitarian

A flexitarian usually eats a plant-based diet but occasionally adds meats to the diet. They are also known as semi-vegetarians.

Fruitarian

This is a veganism subset and it mainly or fully consists of fruits, seeds and nuts. It does not include animal products. The difference with the plant-based diet is that fruitarianism only considers fruits and seeds while a plant-based diet considers other plants as food.

Macrobiotic diet

This diet combines the concepts of principles of certain diets and spirituality of Buddhism to balance physical and spiritual wellness

## The Plant-Based Food Group

Leaves

Leaf vegetables, or greens, are one of the most nutrient-dense foods you can eat. They contain plenty of vitamins (especially K, A, C, and folate) and minerals (like iron, magnesium, and potassium), as well as lots of chlorophyll, which is cleansing to the human system, particularly the liver. If you feel maxed out on salads, try adding some greens to a fruit smoothie or a soup. Puréed greens shrink quite a bit. The wide variety of leaves includes lettuce, kale, spinach, cabbage, Swiss chard, mizuna, arugula, bok choy, collard greens, mustard greens, dandelion greens, endive, escarole, watercress, sorrel, and tatsoi.

Roots

Root vegetables are generally made up of complex carbohydrates and starches. This is why they are usually cooked before being eaten, since cooking breaks down the starch molecules into easier-to-digest forms. However, carrots and radishes are commonly eaten raw in North America. The many root vegetables include carrot, beet, parsnip, rutabaga, turnip, sweet potato, potato, celeriac, and radish. Many root vegetables, such as beets, radishes, and turnips, also have very tasty leaves.

Bulbs

This group includes onions, leeks, and garlic. Garlic's claim to fame is boosting cardiovascular health; it's been shown in many studies to reduce cholesterol, inhibit platelet aggregation (when platelets in the blood stick together, which is how clots form), and reduce blood pressure. Onions are also recommended for cardiovascular health, since they have sulfur compounds similar to the ones that make garlic so powerful.

Stems

Stem vegetables include asparagus, celery, and kohlrabi. They are all very nutritious green vegetables with very few calories. Kohlrabi is a relative of cabbage and broccoli, so it contains the powerful cancer-fighting and anti-inflammatory compounds of this family of vegetables.

Vines

Although some of these vegetables are botanically considered fruit, when it comes to nutrition and cooking, they are in the vegetable category. These vegetables have high water content and will shrink considerably when cooked. Because this category includes a variety of vegetables, they have very different nutritional profiles, but vine veggies are generally rich in carotenoids and vitamin C. Vine vegetables include zucchini, squash, eggplant, cucumber, peas, okra, tomato, and bell and hot peppers.

Flowers

Yes, flowers can also be vegetables! This group includes broccoli, cauliflower, and artichoke. Broccoli, as a dark green vegetable, is packed with nutrients and antioxidants. Although cauliflower has no color, it has similar nutrients and is just as good for you like broccoli.

Mushrooms

Mushrooms are not plants (they are fungi), but nutritionally they get lumped in with vegetables. The difference with mushrooms is that they eat organic matter and do not use photosynthesis like plants. Since they are a totally different organism than other vegetables, they have value in our diet by bringing in different nutrients, such as selenium and copper, as well as a powerful anti-inflammatory, cardioprotective, cancer-protective, and immune-supportive compounds. Mushrooms are high in minerals and protein per calorie and are also a good source of B vitamins.

Some of the mushrooms you might find in your local markets include chanterelle, shiitake, oyster, cremini, button, morel, and puffball. There are also many other types of edible mushrooms, including mushrooms used for their healing powers in Chinese medicine—some powerful enough to combat cancer.

Nuts and Seeds

1.Chia Seeds

Chia seeds are amazing sources of vitamin C, protein, fiber, and calcium. They have to be soaked in liquid and allowed to expand. Once properly prepared, you can sprinkle them on top of almost anything!

2.Pumpkin Seeds

Pumpkin seeds work great for a tasty and easy snack and can also be added to salads, yogurt, and soups. They pack a lot of great nutrients like Vitamins C, E, and K, omega-3 fatty acids, and iron in a small package.

3.Almonds

Commonly considered nuts, almonds are more accurately categorized as a fruit of the almond tree. They are wonderful sources of fiber, protein, magnesium, phosphorus, calcium, potassium, iron, and B vitamins. Like soybeans, they are often used in dairy substitutes and they have been shown to lower cholesterol, strengthen bones, and promote a healthy cardiovascular system. Plus, they are great for your skin and hair!

4.Flaxseeds

Flaxseeds are great additives to plant-based meals. They can be ground up and added to smoothies, oatmeal, cereal, or baked into muffins, bread, and cookies. They are high in protein, magnesium, zinc, and B vitamins. They also aid in digestion and help with weight loss by suppressing appetite.

5.Walnuts

These nuts are some of the best natural sources of omega-3 fatty acids. They also contain plenty of vitamin E, protein, calcium, zinc, and potassium. These, like many of the other nuts and seeds on this list, can be enjoyed alone as a snack or added to other dishes.

6.Sesame Seeds

Sesame seeds are a great natural way to lower cholesterol and high blood pressure and can also help with afflictions like migraines, arthritis, and asthma. They are great in bread and crackers and can be used in stir-fry meals and salads.

7.Sunflower Seeds

These seeds are great for vitamin E and contain healthy fats, B vitamins, and iron. They can be eaten dry and are also used to make butter, a great alternative to dairy.

8.Cashews

Though cashews, like almonds, are not technically nuts and are rather the fruit of the cashew tree, they are most commonly treated as nuts. With their low sodium content and great flavor, they are a popular source of protein and vitamins.

9.Brazil Nuts

These delicious nuts from the Bertholletia excelsa tree mature inside a large coconut-like shell. They are wonderful for protein, fiber, iron, and many B-complex vitamins.

10.Pine Nuts

Pine nuts contain great antioxidants as well as lots of iron, magnesium, and potassium. They are low in calories and go wonderfully with many dishes. You can use them in baked foods or add them in sauces like an Italian pesto.

Legumes

1.Edamame

These cooked soybeans are not only delicious, but they also have an incredible amount of protein. In just one cup, a serving of edamame will give you 18 grams of protein. Look for the certified organic seal, though, because many soybeans in the United States are treated with pesticides or genetically modified. Edamame works great as a stand-alone snack or appetizer and can also be added into meals as a side or in a stir-fry.

2.Lentils

Easy to incorporate into almost any meal in a variety of forms, lentils provide an excellent source of low-calorie and high-fiber protein. They contain 9 grams of protein per half cup serving. They are also incredibly helpful in lowering cholesterol and promoting heart health. You can prepare them as a side dish, use them to make veggie burgers, substitute them for meat and make a delicious taco filling in a slow cooker or make a yummy dip with them.

3.Black Beans

Black beans are another vegetable like lentils that are wonderfully multi-use. They have great fiber, folate, potassium, and vitamin B6. They contain 7.6 grams of protein in every serving and can be used to make anything from veggie burgers to vegan brownies. Imagine that!

4.Potatoes

Potatoes are a great, low-cost source of protein (4 grams per medium potato) and potassium. They're tasty and heart-healthy!

5.Spinach

One of the best green vegetables for protein (3 grams per serving), cooked spinach is an excellent addition to your plant-based diet.

6.Broccoli

When cooked, you get 2 grams per serving of this vegetable and also an excellent dose of fiber.

7.Brussels Sprouts

Another great green vegetable for protein, Brussels sprouts gives you 2 grams of protein per serving alongside a great deal of potassium and vitamin K. Be sure to get the fresh version, though, as they taste a whole lot better than the frozen kind!

8.Lima Beans

Containing 7.3 grams of protein per serving when cooked, lima beans make an amazing side dish or addition to a healthy salad. They also contain leucine, an amino acid that aids in muscle synthesis!

9.Peanuts and Peanut Butter

Widely recognized as a super food by meat-eaters and plant-based eaters alike, peanuts and peanut butter contain 7 grams of protein per serving and can be used in so many different ways. And who doesn't love a good childhood staple PB&J sandwich? Nearly all kinds of peanut butter are vegan, but keep a lookout for any that might contain honey if you are keeping strictly vegan and cutting out all animal products.

10.Chickpeas

Chickpeas are another versatile legume that can be prepared in a multitude of ways. Perhaps the most popular preparation is in the form of delicious hummus. With 6 grams of protein per serving, it'll be hard not to spread it on everything you eat!

Whole Grains

1.Quinoa

Quinoa certainly has made a splash onto the health food scene with countless people boasting about its beneficial qualities. Although it is actually a seed, we treat it mainly as a grain in the way in which it is prepared. This South American gem has an incredible amount of protein and omega-3 fatty acids and is an important staple of anyone looking to get more of these nutrients within a plant-based diet. It can be used in a multitude of dishes and is as versatile as it is healthy!

2.Wheat

A classic staple, whole wheat is incredibly beneficial to your health. Each serving of whole grain has about 2 to 3 grams of fiber, which is a great way to make sure your body is functioning healthily and properly. Be sure to steer clear of multi-grain, however, and go for the stuff marked 100% whole grain to make sure you are getting exactly what you need!

3.Oats

These whole grains are packed full of heart-healthy antioxidants. Oats are great and can be enjoyed as a fulfilling breakfast in the form of oatmeal and they can also be ground up and used as a healthier flour substitute when baking. Unsweetened oats are the best to buy and if you are craving a little something sugary, throw in a few berries or a dollop of honey if you wish.

4.     Brown Rice

Brown rice is incredibly high in antioxidants and good vitamins. It is relative, white rice is far less beneficial as much of these healthy nutrients get destroyed during the process of milling. You can also opt for red and black rice or wild rice. The meal options for this healthy grain are limitless!

5.Rye

Rye is an amazing whole grain that contains four times the fiber of regular whole wheat and gives you almost 50% of day-to-day recommended iron intake. When shopping for rye, however, be sure to look for the whole rye marking as a lot of what is on the market is made with refined flour, thus cutting the benefits in half.

6.Barley

This whole grain is a miracle food for lowering high cholesterol. It can be quick-cooked like oats and serves as a delicious side dish. You can add whatever kind of toppings you desire to give it your own personal flair! Be sure again to seek out the whole-grain barley as other types may have the bran or germ removed.

7.Buckwheat

Buckwheat is a great gluten-free grain option for those with celiac disease or gluten intolerance. It's a great source of magnesium and manganese. Buckwheat is used to make delicious gluten free pancakes and easily becomes a morning staple!

8.Bulgur

This grain is a truly excellent source of iron and magnesium. It also contains a wonderful amount of protein and fiber with one cup containing about 75% of daily recommended fiber and 25% or daily recommended protein. It goes great in salads and soups and is easy to cook. Talk about amazing!

9.Couscous

This grain is another great source of fiber. A lot of the couscous you see in the store will be made from refined flour, though, so you must seek out the whole wheat kind so that you can get all the healthy, yummy benefits.

10.Corn

Whole corn is a fantastic source of phosphorus, magnesium, and B vitamins. It also promotes healthy digestion and contains heart-healthy antioxidants. It is important to seek out organic corn in order to bypass all of the genetically modified product that is out on the market.

Fruits

1.Avocado

Widely acknowledged as an incredibly beneficial and healthy super-fruit, avocados truly are miracle fruits.

They are the best way possible to get the kind of substantial serving of healthy monounsaturated fatty acids that many people subscribing to a plant-based diet seek to supplement. They also contain about 20 different vitamins and minerals and are packed with important nutrients. On top of that, they taste amazing and go well with almost any dish, breakfast, lunch, or dinner!

2.Grapefruit

Grapefruits are packed full of Vitamin C, containing much more than oranges. Half a grapefruit provides you with almost 50% of your recommended daily vitamin C. It also gives you incredible levels of Vitamin A, fiber, and potassium. It can help with afflictions like arthritis and is a great remedy for oily skin.

3.Pineapple

This fruit can be prepared and enjoyed in a variety of ways making it not only a tasty and fun treat but also a great healthy choice! It is full of anti-inflammatory nutrients that can help reduce the risk of stroke or heart attack. Some studies show that it also increases fertility.

4.Blueberries

These little berries not only taste delicious and go with so many different dishes, but they are also full of vitamin C and healthful antioxidants. Studies also show that it promotes eye health and can slow macular degeneration, which causes older adults to go blind.

5.Pomegranate

Whether in juice form or seed, consuming pomegranate is a great way to get potassium. It has fantastic antioxidants (three times more than green tea or red wine) that work to promote cardiovascular and heart health as well as lower cholesterol levels

6.Apple

The old saying "an apple a day keeps the doctor away" is not just an old wife' tale! It is low-calorie and incredibly healthy. Apples contain antioxidants that protect brain cell health and are heart-healthy. They can also lower high cholesterol and aid in weight loss and healthy teeth.

7.Kiwi

This tart, delicious fruit is not only unique but also full of great vitamins like C and E. These are powerful antioxidants that some studies show help with eye health and can even lower the chances of cancer. They are low-calorie and very high in fiber. This makes them great for aiding in weight loss and they make a wonderful, quick, easy, and guilt-free snack.

8.Mango

Mangoes have excellent levels of the nutrient beta-carotene. The body converts this into Vitamin A which in turn strengthens bone health and the immune system. They also have a huge amount of Vitamin C- 50% of the daily recommended value to be exact.

9.Lemons

Everyone knows that lemons and other citrus fruit are high in Vitamin C, however, they are also an excellent source of antioxidants, fiber, and folate. Lemons can help lower cholesterol, the risk of some kinds of cancer, and blood pressure. All at just 17 calories a serving!

10.Cranberries

Cranberries are another fruit that has more than one health benefit. They have great vitamin C and fiber levels and have more antioxidants than many other fruits and vegetables. At only 45 calories a serving, it is a great way to boost your immune system, keep your urinary tract healthy, and absorb other important nutrients like Vitamins E, K, and manganese.

Spices and Herbs

Spices and herbs are not only a way to add rich flavor to your dishes but they also have small amounts of important nutrients. A study of vegetarian males eating an Indian diet showed that they got between 3.9 and 7.9 percent of their essential amino acid requirements, along with about 6 percent of calcium and 4 percent of iron, just from the seasonings in their food.

Many spices have protein, and although it doesn't amount to much in terms of grams, it provides a source of some of the amino acids that may be low in plant foods. Popular spices that will add a world of flavor to your food include cumin, coriander, cinnamon, paprika, and nutmeg.

Herbs like parsley, cilantro, mint, ginger, and basil pack loads of nutrients, and are most beneficial and flavorful when you eat them fresh. Parsley gives women 22 percent of their daily vitamin C recommendation, and men 27 percent, in just 4 tablespoons. All fresh herbs, like leafy greens, have a high antioxidant and chlorophyll content, providing energy and helping your body neutralize free radicals.

## Nutrients in Plant-Based Diet
Carbohydrates

Some people worry about consuming too many carbohydrates by eating plant foods. Carbohydrates are your body's main source of energy and are completely healthy if you eat them in the form of whole foods (such as whole grains, vegetables, and fruit), since they contain lots of vitamins, minerals, antioxidants, water, and fiber. Fiber is also a carbohydrate, but its role is to facilitate digestion rather than give energy.

Whole grains and fruit have the highest levels of carbohydrates, with about 70 to 90 percent carbohydrate content. Eating a banana is an instant energy boost. The best food sources of fiber are psyllium or flaxseed and leafy green vegetables.

Protein

Protein can be found in all cells of the body. It helps to repair and build muscles, skin, bones, and the immune system. Protein is also needed to create hormones and enzymes, which are made up of amino acids. The body can make some of the amino acids but definitely not all of them. The ones the body can't make are called essential amino acids and must come from the foods you eat. Eating mostly plant-based foods can meet your body's daily protein needs.

Protein is an essential nutrient in the body. It not only helps in building and repairing muscles, but it also aids in maintaining our skin and bone health. The immune system also requires protein to function optimally in warding off diseases. So, if you are new to a vegan diet, you may have questions concerning your protein sources. Of course, this is attributed to the myth that plant-based diets don't provide the body with sufficient nutrients.

However, several plant foods will provide you with the protein you need in your diet. Some of these foods include beans, soy products, seeds, nuts, peas, vegetables, and whole grains. When looking for proteins in vegetables, your shopping cart should be filled with veggies like broccoli, yellow sweet corn, potatoes, lentils, green peas, Brussels sprouts, broccoli rabe, avocado, and cauliflower.

Evidently, you can see that you have plenty of options to choose from when in search of protein in your diet. Now, let's do some math to determine the amount of protein you might need in your diet. According to the Dietary Reference Intakes, the amount of protein you should consume daily is equivalent to 0.8 grams per kilogram of your body weight, or 0.36 grams per pound. Say you weigh 80 kilograms. You should multiply this by 0.8 grams to determine the protein quantity you require daily. In this case, the quantity of protein will be 64 grams.

The various foods mentioned above offer varying amounts of protein. This implies that combining several veggies together will provide you with what you need. A one cup serving of lentils, for instance, will provide you with 18 grams of protein. A cup of green peas, on the other hand, will only provide you with 8.5 grams of protein. Judging from the numbers, all you need is a mix of different plant foods to meet your daily protein intake.

Fats

Your body needs enough dietary fat to function, maintain metabolism, and absorb and utilize minerals and certain vitamins. People with cold hands and feet, amenorrhea (missed menstrual periods), or dry skin, hair, or throat may need more fats in their diet, and particularly saturated fats like coconut oil. To be clear, eating healthy fat in reasonable amounts doesn't make you fat.

Oils are 100 percent fat and aren't something you necessarily need to eat, but they are great for carrying rich flavor and mouthfeel in a dish, particularly when you're transitioning to a healthier diet. If you use oils, it's best to keep them minimal and use unrefined oils like olive, coconut, sesame, and avocado. (Refined oils include canola, soy, sunflower, and corn oil.) You can easily sauté vegetables for two people with just a teaspoon of oil.

That doesn't mean you should never eat oils, though, and some people can actually benefit from concentrated fats. For example, flax oil or concentrated DHA might be necessary for someone with issues digesting and utilizing omega-3 fatty acids.

Omega-3 fatty acids are also essential nutrients, meaning that the body cannot produce them. There are three forms of omega-3 fatty acids:

Docosahexaenoic acid (DHA)

Alpha-linolenic acid (ALA)

Eicosapentaenoic acid (EPA)

Individuals who eat fish usually obtain DHA and EPA. ALA, on the other hand, is obtained from plant foods. The good news is that the body can convert ALA obtained from plants into DHA and EPA. However, the process is not as efficient. Consequently, you could supplement your diet with hemp seed oil, flaxseed oil, or chia seeds to aid in optimizing the conversion process.

Other recommended foods to ingest include algal oil, walnuts, perilla oil, and Brussels sprouts.

The information detailed in this section should help you realize that important nutrients that are often assumed to be present only in animal products can also be obtained from plant foods. Therefore, knowing and understanding the nutrients you are getting from your plant foods is important; it confirms that you are getting all the vital nutrients your body requires for optimal functioning.

Vitamin C

Vitamin C will be an easier nutrient to obtain since most fruits and vegetables can provide the body with this vital nutrient. This vitamin helps in strengthening the body's immune system. As a result, vitamin C is often perceived as a remedy for the common cold. Recommended vegan foods to add to your diet here include broccoli, pineapple, Brussels.

# Chapter 3 Calories Tables And Description Of Plant-based Foods And Micronutrients

Plants are rich in micronutrients that come from the soil they grow in, the basics of life they need to grow, the phytochemicals they use to protect themselves, attract insects and adapt to the changes around them.  As plants are unable to move as animals do, they have a uniquely full tool chest of macro and micro-nutrients that enable them to adapt to the changing environment around them.  These micronutrients are just as valuable to humans as they are to the plants but in different ways. Below is a breakdown of the basic micronutrients found in fruits, vegetables, nuts, seeds, and legumes.

Vitamins

Vibrant vegetables and fruits are a dense source of vitamins that are essential to overall health and wellness.

Vitamin A: Also known as beta-carotene is a carotenoid found in yellow, orange and dark green fruits and veg, most notably carrots, spinach, and broccoli.  It protects against infections and is essential for eye and skin health.

Vitamin B: This group of vitamins is responsible for maintaining the nervous system and cognitive function, DNA and blood cell production.

1 is responsible for nervous system health and aids in the breakdown and absorption of food.  Found in peas, whole grains, and most fruits and vegetables.

2 is responsible for energy production and healthy skin and eyes and found in asparagus, spinach, and broccoli.

3 is great for healthy skin and energy production and is found in peanuts, avocados, peas, and mushrooms.

6 is also essential for energy production and is found in chickpeas, potatoes, banana, squash, and nuts.

9 is also known as folate and is essential for fetal development and growth and healthy cell division.  It is found in legumes, asparagus, spinach, arugula, kale, and beets.

12 is predominantly sourced from animal products but you can find it in some organic soy products but most notably nutritional yeast.

Vitamin C: An essential vitamin important for cell growth and energy production as well as tissue repair and wound healing.  It is one of the most powerful antioxidants and is found in strawberries, spinach, Brussel sprouts, sweet potatoes, and tomatoes.

Vitamin E: A powerful antioxidant that protects the body from free radical damage including premature aging.  It's of great support to the immune system, protecting it against external pathogens.  It is found in sunflower seeds, almonds, hazelnuts, spinach, and broccoli.

Vitamin K: This vitamin plays a major role in the clotting cascade and also in bone health.  It is found in all green leafy veg as well as cruciferous veg and green tea.

Minerals

Macro-minerals:  we need these in large quantities from our diet.

Calcium: This essential mineral plays roles in bone, heart, muscle and nerve health.  Foods high in calcium are spinach, collard greens, seeds, almonds, soybeans, and butter beans.

Chloride: This mineral plays a part in body fluid balance including digestive juices.  It is found in sea salt, tomatoes, lettuce, celery, and rye bread.

Magnesium: This mineral regulates blood sugar and assists in energy production.  It also helps your muscles, kidneys, bones and heart function effectively.  It is found in spinach, quinoa, dark chocolate, almonds, avocado, and black beans.

Phosphorous:  This mineral is found in bones and works with calcium in maintaining healthy mineral balance within the body.  It is found in pumpkin, sunflower seeds, lentils, chickpeas, oatmeal, and quinoa.

Sodium: The current population gets excess sodium from all pre-packaged foods and restaurant meals, so there is no need to go looking for extra sodium in the diet.

Potassium: This mineral is essential in blood pressure balance, muscle health, and nerve function.  It is found in avocado, bananas, apricots, grapefruit, potatoes, mushrooms, cucumbers and zucchini.

Trace Minerals: We just need tiny amounts of these from our foods.

Copper: Essential in the formation of red blood cells and iron absorption.  It is found in whole grains, beans, potatoes, cocoa, black pepper, and dark leafy greens.

Cobalt:  This trace mineral works closely with B12 in the formation of hemoglobin.  It is found in nuts, broccoli, oats, and spinach.

Manganese:  Plays many roles in enzyme activity and cellular level antioxidants.  It is found in pineapple, peanuts, brown rice, spinach, sweet potato, pecans, and green tea.

Iodine: Essential for thyroid function, you can find it in seaweed, lima beans, and prunes.

Iron: Used to make hemoglobin and as a carrier for essential nutrients in the blood.  In plant form, it is found in cashews, spinach, whole grains, tofu, potatoes, and lentils.

Selenium: A trace mineral essential in the role of reproduction, DNA production, and antioxidant function. It is found in brazil nuts, lentils, cashew nuts, and potatoes.

Zinc: As your body doesn't store zinc, it needs to be consumed daily because it plays important roles in nutrient metabolism, immune system maintenance, and enzyme function. It is found in legumes, nuts, seeds, potatoes, kale and green beans.

Colors

The colors in fruits and vegetables point to what kinds of nutrients they contain.

White foods: Contain sulfur and can have anti-cancer properties. Found in cauliflower, garlic, leeks, and onions.

Green foods: Contain lutein and vitamin K. Found in dark leafy greens, broccoli, avocado.

Purple foods: Contain anthocyanins, which are powerful antioxidants. Found in blueberries, eggplant, red cabbage, and blackberries.

Red foods: Contain lycopene and has therapeutic properties for the heart. Found in strawberries, watermelon, tomatoes, and red bell peppers.

# Chapter 4 The Plant-based Diet Meal Plan (starting Meal Plan)

Plant-based meal arranging is somewhat more confused in the first place contrasted with simply preparing up arbitrary meals. Things being what they are, the reason the hell would it be a good idea for you to try and trouble and instruct yourself on the best way to meal plan appropriately? All things considered, it can offer you a larger number of advantages than you may suspect.

How Would You Like:

A complain free week

Less basic leadership and overthinking meals

Easier shopping and a lower grocery bill

Effortlessly adhering to sound propensities

Easily meeting individual healthful needs

Trying new recipes

Having an arrangement for your weight loss or weight gain

Knowing what works best for you

Keeping yourself responsible by having every one of the fixings and meals close by

Beginning Tips

Before we're getting directly into the vegan meat of the issue, there are a couple of tips to think about that can make your meal arranging venture significantly simpler, less startling, and substantially more energizing! We truly need you to succeed and this implies you're getting a charge out of the procedure just as the outcomes here.

Step by step instructions to Do It

Try not to Spend All Day on Meal Prepping

Except if you need to get worn out or meal prep is your obsession. Pull out all the stops! Something else, set a clock for two hours and when it dings you are DONE! That is sufficient opportunity to prep veggies, vegetables, cook grains, and select recipes if necessary. Make the most of your end of the week! Try not to do a lot without a moment's delay. You'll be astounded at what you can achieve in two centered hours.

Make An Arrangement

Put aside 45 minutes or thereabouts and select your recipes for the week. Spare them on your telephone by taking a screen capture or spare them on a Pinterest board or go old fashioned and print them out! Simply keep them somewhere sheltered! This guide allows you 30 days of recipes for breakfast, lunch, and dinner, so you have the opportunity to build up a framework that works for you going ahead!

Set aside Cash

Shop the deals in the Sunday paper. (Truly, this is as yet a thing!) Select your week by week recipes as indicated by what you can purchase for less! Verify what grocery stores in your general vicinity twofold coupons. You can spare a TON along these lines and no; you don't need to be an outrageous coupon to do it! Spare huge internet shopping by utilizing applications like Ebates and ibotta. Their costs are up to half off – everyday – and – they convey!

Use Multi-Purpose Recipes

Discover recipes you can twofold or you realize will consider scraps you can have for lunch. You know, Monday night's bean stew transforms into Tuesday's Taco sort of thing! I've incorporated a few multi-reason plant-based recipes beneath on the off chance that you're intrigued. See bean stew, soups, and [vegan] burgers.

Cluster Cook

Concoct a major cluster of entire grains like dark colored rice, quinoa, or grain to go with your week by week meals on Saturday or Sunday. Douse and cook chickpeas and beans on your favored meal prep day. At that point portion them out for plates of mixed greens, buddha bowls, and bean stews. This procedure won't take up your whole day, yet it will spare you huge amounts of time later in the week!

Try not to Get Too Gourmet

Start with straightforward recipes and develop your direction. Start with simple recipes!

Picking Your Food

There are a lot of interesting points when picking the nourishments which you will incorporate into your meal plan. Once more, remember these to make the procedure progressively charming and fun! Along these lines, for your plant-based meal arranging, ensure you...

Go for the nourishments you effectively like before purchasing an immense sack of Brussel's sprouts or rhubarb

Use what you have at home to set aside cash and abstain from squandering any nourishment

Keep a running rundown of what you need so you won't overlook anything and remain well-supplied

Make a grocery rundown to go out on the town to shop each week

Go for mass areas and occasional produce to set aside some cash

Look out for solidified or pre-cut/pre-destroyed produce and canned vegetables to make your life simpler

Next, stock up your kitchen! By what other methods would you have the option to browse a decent assortment of delicious, solid, and adaptable nourishments to use in your meal plan?

Additional tip: Have an unfaltering stock of snacks in the house, for example, fruit, nuts, and wafers!

## Planning The Plant-based Meal

Since you've found out about the absolute most significant establishments, we can get into the arranging it-hard and fast part. When thinking of an idea for a meal plan, we like to concentrate on the accompanying rules. Check whether your nourishment or meals are:

Nutrient thick

Low in included fat, salt and sugar

Rich in fiber

Filling and fulfilling

Based on starches

Adequate to meet your caloric and nourishing needs

This may appear to be somewhat unique to you at the present time, so we needed to give you an understanding of what your meals ought to resemble. When taking a gander at the distinctive nourishment classes, here are the means by which you could make sweet or flavorful balanced vegan meals.

Breakfast Blueprint

Pick at least one of every classification - for cutting edge plant munchers, don't hesitate to include a few vegetables like spinach or solidified cauliflower to your smoothies.

Starches

Oats, bread, grain, hash tans, flapjacks

Fruit

New, dried, solidified, for example, berries, apples, bananas

Vegetables

Soy milk, soy yogurt, tofu (for scramble), nutty spread

Nuts and Seeds

Flaxseeds, chia seeds, pecans, almond spread
Lunch and Dinner Blueprint

Once more, pick one or a few instances of every class - relying upon your vitality or weight objectives, you can join more vegetables or nuts.

Additional items

Nuts, seeds, nut or seed margarine, fruit, sauces, spices, condiments

With respect to snacks, there are no fixed principles – simply do whatever it takes not to utilize this season of day to sneak some garbage or candy machine nourishment into your eating regimen. Some better thoughts are crisp fruit, dried fruit, nuts, entire grain wafers, rice cakes, hummus, veggie sticks, cooked chickpeas, granola bars, sans oil popcorn, or just a few scraps.

You may be thinking now: "Yet in what capacity will I meet the entirety of my wholesome needs on the off chance that I don't generally follow my nourishment? Isn't that difficult on a plant-based eating routine?" This next part is for you to teach yourself and facilitate your brain.

Nutrients and Foods to Focus On

It is great to begin by saying that an entire nourishments plant-based eating routine is just about the most nutrient-thick diet you could think of. That being stated, there are still approaches to pass up a couple of basic ones in the event that you don't concentrate on a decent assortment of nourishments. A few people like to simply eat a lot of fruit or starches, overlooking vegetables and seeds for instance.

It's not actually simpler for individuals on an omnivorous eating routine to meet the entirety of their wholesome needs since they normally get too little fiber, nutrients, and minerals while having an excess of immersed fat and cholesterol. In this way, everybody ought to design their eating regimen astutely!

Concerning the couple of nutrients that are somewhat harder to jump on an absolutely plant-based eating routine, here are the best sources to go for and incorporate into your everyday diet. Pick in any event one for every nutrient:

Calcium: strengthened soy milk, tofu, kale, broccoli, vegetables, sesame, entire wheat

Iron: vegetables, tofu, tomato sauce, dull green vegetables, oats, quinoa, darker rice

Zinc: pumpkin seeds, vegetables, entire grains, verdant green vegetables

Omega-3: flaxseed, chia seeds, pecans, romaine lettuce

Vitamin B12: supplements, strengthened nourishment

Vitamin D: daylight, a few mushrooms, strengthened nourishments, supplements

Portions and Calories

You may even now be pondering about the amount to eat on a plant-based eating regimen. In case you're not mindful of your everyday suggested vitality consumption, check your BMR and include your movement level utilizing a straightforward number cruncher. Most adults need around at any rate 2000 calories for every day which you shouldn't attempt to undermine excessively, in any event, when attempting to get in shape.

Plant-based nourishments, particularly when entire and natural, have a lower calorie thickness which means you should eat bigger portions and it will be significantly simpler to lose some weight in light of the fact that these nourishments include considerably more mass.

If you wind up excessively stuffed or too hungry following a day of eating, make a note and modify in like manner the following day or at whatever point you're making your new meal plan. We can't disclose to you precisely the amount you have to eat, so please have your age, sex, action level, anxiety, and wellbeing status at the top of the priority list. We're advocates for eating naturally, which means go get something when you're ravenous and quit chomping when you're easily full. It's on you to choose what number of meals every day you'd like to eat and if you need to snack. Various things work for various individuals here. Regardless of if it's 2, 3, 4, or 5 little meals for each day – work with your inclinations and your calendar.

Redoing for Weight Goals

When altering your meal plan to your needs and objectives, we prompt that you move your concentration starting with one nutrition type then onto the next and not to remove something totally. All entire plant-based nourishments are gainful to your wellbeing (insofar as you're not prejudiced or oversensitive to them) and can be eaten. We're working with the guideline of calorie thickness here which you can use to either lose, gain, or keep up your weight while powering your body with sound nourishments.

In case you're into weight picking up or lifting weights, center more around entire flour items and vegetables just as nuts, seeds, and dried fruit to get enough calories. The equivalent goes for individuals with a little craving who battle with eating enough. You may likewise need to incorporate more smoothies and even squeezes into your eating routine to build your calories. Go simple on enormous crude servings of mixed greens and vegetable stews since they offer just barely any calories while including a great deal of mass. Similarly, in case you're into weight loss, center around non-boring vegetables to go with your entire, flawless starches like potatoes or dark colored rice for lunch and dinner. Try not to decrease the starches excessively, have around half vegetables and starches on your plate. Go simple on flour items and dried fruit, have crisp fruit as a snack and attempt to eat a green serving of mixed greens each day. Likewise, keep away from included oils and lessen the measure of nuts and seeds you devour.

# Chapter 5 The Plant-based Diet Meal Plan

In contrary to the popular belief, transitioning to a plant-based diet is quite easy, if you take the right steps at the right time. By switching to a diet that includes more fibers, vitamins and minerals and avoiding meat and dairy products, you are not depriving yourself from any necessary nutrients. In fact, you are taking a step towards health improvement and a better life in general. Following this 4-week program for transitioning to a plant-based diet will get you the results you wanted, which are healthy eating habits and the ability to enjoy food like you always did.

What is important to know when starting to transition to a plant-based diet is that this process should be done gradually. You should by no means drop meat and dairy ingredients right away and strictly force yourself to eat plant-based foods. The point of this program is to make your transition easy and effortless by gradually creating habits that are going to lead to a full transition without craving to return to your old eating habits. So, take it easy, step by step, and let's get into it!

## Week 1

At the very beginning of your transition journey, you are going to start learning which foods to turn to and which ingredients to leave behind. The key here is to take things slowly, which is why in the first week you should focus on your breakfasts. Your meal plan for this week is going to consist of your regular meals with a bit of adjustments done to them. As this is the first stage of your plant-based diet transition process, you need to start balancing your usual diet with the changes you are about to introduce to it. For the beginning, go through the contents of your refrigerator and try to take out as many animal products as possible. Stock your refrigerator with plant-based ingredients to start your transition process! Foods you should be bringing into your fridge include berries, cabbage, broccoli, kale, beans, etc. Also, when choosing your ingredients, look for good quality and check the origin of the products, as you don't want anything processed to find a way to your kitchen.

Don't feel like you need to start avoiding meat and other animal foods right away. There should be no pressure to do so, as this is a calm and slow diet transition. In week 1 we are going to attack your breakfast habits while the rest of your meals of the day are going to stay the same.

To help prepare yourself for the second week of your transition process, try to balance your plate by adding more plant-based ingredients than you used to. The more you increase your whole foods intake at this stage of the transition, the easier it is going to be to adjust to what the second, third and fourth week has to offer! Therefore, in week 1, your goal is to switch to plant-based breakfasts with fiber and high nutritional value. Here are three breakfast recipes for you to get inspired to start changing your morning meal habits.

#1 Three Minutes Oatmeal

Ingredients:

1/2 cup of oats

1 ripe banana

1 teaspoon of cinnamon

1 teaspoon of grounded flax seeds

½ cup of water

½ cup of plant-based milk (soy/ rice/ almond/ hemp)

Toppings of choice (peanut butter/ fresh fruit/ frozen berries/ seeds/ nuts)

Directions:

Roast the oats, flax seeds together with cinnamon on a preheated non-stick pan for about 30 seconds. Add water and milk - start with little and rather add more to reach your desired consistency. Shortly before finishing, add sliced ripe banana (spotted), that is going to serve as a substitute for a sweetener.

Use this recipe as a base on how to prepare oatmeal and try to experiment with other ingredients such as frozen berries, nut butter, cacao, spices (turmeric), nuts or seeds. Mix those ingredients into the oatmeal either while cooking or only when serving as a topping.

Remember that you are trying to avoid processed foods. Therefore, do not forget to read the labels when purchasing your ingredients. Peanut butter should have only one ingredient - peanuts. You do not want any added salt, oil or sugar. The same is valid for dried fruits and plant-based milk (avoid added sugar). It is simple, just read the ingredients of the products.

#2 Overnight Oats

Ingredients:

½ cup of oats

½ cup of nuts or seeds of choice (walnuts, hazelnuts, sunflower seeds, pumpkin seeds, ...)

Dried fruit of choice (resins, cranberries, dates)

Directions:

Do you want to prepare your breakfast the night before and not lose time in the morning? Just mix all the ingredients together and simply soak them overnight. In the morning just pour the excess water away and breakfast is served. If desired you can add some fresh fruit.

Soaking oats, nuts and seeds makes them easier digestible. It also wakes up a different taste in them, that you might have not experienced before.

#3 Green Smoothie

Smoothie is a good breakfast when you want to start your day quickly and right away with a bunch of nutrients. The beauty of a smoothie is that you can add ingredients that you otherwise have problems adding to your diet. Perfect examples are greens such as spinach or kale.

For beginners, green smoothies might be quite a challenge. Therefore, I recommend starting with adding just a small portion of greens and slowly increase the amount over time as you get used to the taste.

Generally, the best basis for a smoothie are bananas as they make the smoothie nicely thick and naturally sweet. Always make sure that your fruits are ripe as fruit in that form is the easiest to digest. Ripe bananas are easy to recognize - the color is yellow (not green) with black spots.

Ingredients:

2 ripe bananas

1 cup fresh baby spinach

1 cup frozen berries

1 cup of water or plant-based milk

Directions:

First fill the blender with greens, then bananas or other fruits of your choice and liquid (water or plant-based milk). Blend until smooth.

## Week 2

In the second week of your transition to a plant-based diet you should be used to eating whole foods and plant-based ingredients for breakfast. Now we are going to step things up and introduce those ingredients to your lunch meals. Therefore, the second week of the program is going to consist of both breakfast and lunch meals made without animal products or any kinds of processed ingredients. You should focus on eliminating dairy products from your lunch meals as well as in general. There's no need to worry about calcium and other nutrients necessary for bone health, as you can get those from healthier plant-based sources as well.

As the second week progresses, you will start learning how to effectively plan your meals and stay on track with your meal plans throughout the week. Dedicate a few minutes every Sunday to creating a meal plan for the following week. This way, you won't run out of ideas for breakfast, lunch or dinner for each day of the week. However, for now, we are only focusing on breakfast and lunch. Therefore, prepare to ditch animal food and combine plant-based ingredients into your lunch meals as well! Here are three recipes to get you started.

#1 Tortilla Pizza

Ingredients:

Tortilla (optimally wholegrain)

Tomato sauce or tomato paste

Vegetable of choice as toppings (suggestion: sliced tomato, corn, garlic, red onion, ...)

Herbs and spices (oregano, garlic powder)

Nutritional yeast (optional)

Directions:

Preheat your oven to 200°C.

If you are using bought tomato sauce then, as always, don't forget to check the ingredients. Make sure the sauce is not high in salt (the salt intake should not exceed 1 gram for 100 gram of the sauce) and that all ingredients are plant based: no cheese, meat or eggs.

If you decided to make your own sauce, also check the package of the tomato paste for the salt intake. Place the paste on a pan and add a little bit of water as the paste itself is thick already. When using this sauce for pizza I would recommend keeping it rather thicker. However, you can use the same sauce as a pasta sauce. In that case water it down. Add a teaspoon of dried oregano and a teaspoon of garlic powder. You might also want to add some chili if you prefer spicy food. If you want to add a bit of cheesy flavor to the sauce mix in also a tablespoon of nutritional yeast. You can also sprinkle the whole pizza with nutritional yeast once it is ready to be baked.

As your sauce is ready, spread it on a tortilla like you would do on a pizza dough. Now is the time to get creative with your favorite pizza toppings. If you want to top it with basil leaves or some greens, I recommend doing so only after the baking process as the leaves would burn in the oven.

To bake your pizza faster, and for more crunchy results, do not use baking tin and only bake the pizza on the grate.

Lower the temperature of the oven to 180°C and bake the pizza for approximately 15 minutes until the crust turns brown.

#2 Baked Sweet Potatoes with Avocado-Beans salad

Ingredients:

1 big or 2 small sweet potatoes

½ of an avocado

½ can of red beans

1 cup fresh spinach

1 tomato

Pepper, salt (optional)

Directions:

Preheat the oven to 250°C. Wash the sweet potatoes and poke a few holes in them using a knife to fasten the baking process. Place the potatoes on a baking paper in the oven, lower the temperature to 200°C and bake for about 40 to 60 minutes. The baking time is always dependent on your oven. Sweet potatoes are fully baked once sugar is running out of them and they are fork tender.

Meanwhile you have time to prepare your filling. Mash one half of an avocado in a bowl, add beans, diced tomato, pepper (freshly grounded if possible) and optionally salt and mix it all together. In general, try to slowly leave out salt from your diet - especially table salt. Don't worry; your taste buds quickly adapt to new tastes and you will not miss added salt in your meals after a short period of time.   If you are not ready to leave out table salt out of your diet, substitute it rather with sea salt or pink Himalayan salt.

Once the potatoes are baked, cut them open. Mash the inside with a fork and create space for the filling. Add spinach leaves first and the avocado mixture on the top. Enjoy!

As with every dish in this book, try not to get stuck with a certain recipe. I would like to give you a guideline for the beginning. Moreover, I would like to encourage you to be creative. Nobody says you cannot add paprika next time instead of tomato, chickpeas instead of red beans or hummus instead of avocado. Remember you are adapting a new lifestyle, not just dieting for 4 weeks.

#3 Red Lentil Soup

Ingredients:

1 cup red lentils

4 cups of water or low- sodium veggie broth

1 table spoon olive oil

1 large carrot (diced)

1 large onion (diced)

1 ½ teaspoon of grounded cardamom

½ teaspoon of salt

Black pepper

Juice of 1 lemon

Directions:

Heat olive oil in a big pot. Add onion and cardamom, salt and little bit of black pepper and stir until the onion turns little brown. Add lentils and carrots and stir to combine. In this time, the soup is getting its most flavor, so spend a few minutes constantly mixing it, so it doesn't burn at the bottom.

Finally add water or veggie broth (4 cups for each cup of lentils), cover the pot and let it cook on low heat for about 15- 20 minutes.

How do you recognize if it's done? Firstly, when tasting the lentils. Red lentils are falling apart while cooking. Therefore, they should be melting in your mouth when tasting. Secondly, check the carrots with stabbing a piece with a knife. Once the piece slides down the knife, the carrot is cooked. In case it sticks on the knife, keep cooking. This rule generally counts for coking any kind of root vegetable.

When finished cooking, add freshly squeezed lemon juice. Mix it all in and enjoy.

You can keep the soup refrigerated for 5 days. However, it is going to thicken with every day, so you can either water it down or keep it as it is and use it as sauce to be eaten with rice, couscous, quinoa or bread.

Are you enjoying the recipes so far?

## Week 3

In week three you are going to switch your dinner meals to the plant-based diet, that is, use only plant-based ingredients to prepare your food. With the third week, you are already wrapping up the transition, as you are now used to your new breakfast and lunch meal strategies. All it takes now is to start implementing those strategies to your dinner meals. At this point, you should already be feeling the improvement in your life caused by starting to transition to a plant-based diet.

With numerous recipes and tips, making plant-based meals is quick and easy, yet as delicious and healthy as you can imagine! In your week three of the transition process you are already near the end of it. What's left to do is introduce these changes to your dinner meals as well and in that way, wrap up a completely new meal plan you are going to be creating every Sunday to stay on track with what you're eating! Here are some delicious and easy plant-based dinner recipes!

#1 Bulgur Salad

Ingredients:

½ cup bulgur wheat

Diced vegetable of your choice (paprika, celery, tomatoes)

½ cup chickpeas

1 cup spinach (diced)

½ avocado

Pepper, salt, oregano, powdered garlic

Directions:

There are two options how to prepare bulgur. If you need to prepare your dish quickly, then simply cook bulgur (1 cup bulgur for 2 cups cold water) in a pot. Bring to a boil, cover the pot and let simmer for 12-15 minutes until tender.

Another option is to soak the bulgur before. Ideally, overnight, but already an hour is enough. Strain it afterwards, rinse one more time and you're good to go. The soaked version tastes lighter and refreshing.

Mash an avocado in a bowl and combine with bulgur. Add in chickpeas and prepared vegetables diced on small pieces. Finally add in seasonings according to your taste.

Give it a final mix and enjoy!

#2 Almond noodles

Ingredients:

100 g of whole grain spaghetti

½ cup of almond butter

¼ cup of water

¼ cup of rice vinegar

2 tablespoons of low sodium soy sauce or tamari

2 tablespoons of Thai red curry paste

Chopped fresh cilantro

Directions:

To prepare this nutrient rich and flavorful dish, cook the spaghetti as you regularly would, while, in the meantime, mix the almond butter, rice vinegar, water, soy sauce or tamari and the Thai red curry paste and whisk it together in a large bowl. Once the spaghetti is cooked, add it into the sauce and mix it together. Serve the meal with the chopped cilantro on top and enjoy!

#3 Pumpkin Soup

Ingredients:

500 g pumpkin (without seeds)

3 cloves garlic (unpeeled)

1 table spoon olive oil

Pepper (amount depending on your own taste)

½ teaspoon Turmeric

Salt (optional)

Cayenne pepper, chili (optional)

Boiled water or low- sodium veggie broth

Directions:

Preheat your oven to 200°C.

Remove the pumpkin seeds and cut the pumpkin to pieces about 2 inches big. Mix them in a bowl together with garlic cloves, olive oil, pepper, turmeric, salt if needed and if you like spicy food you can also add cayenne pepper or chili powder.

Spread prepared pumpkin on a baking tin with baking sheet (moisturize the baking tin, so the baking sheet sticks on it), place the tin in the oven. Lover its temperature to 180°C and bake for about 40 minutes.

Once done, the pumpkin will be fork tender.

Finally place the mixture in a blender (or pot when using submersible blender). Do not forget to free the garlic cloves from its peel. Add two cups of boiled water or veggie broth and blend it all together. Keep adding liquid to achieve the desired thickness of your soup.

Finally, you can always add more spices or salt, if you feel like the soup still needs more taste.

To mix up the recipe, replace the pumpkin with carrots or sweet potatoes. As always, be creative and have fun!

## Week 4

In the final stage of the transition process you should already be used to the new eating habits you've developed. You have switched your breakfast, lunch and dinner meals to plant-based meals but the journey doesn't end there! You still have got a lot to learn, from how to combat cravings to how to make some of the most delicious plant-based meals ever! To combat your cravings, increase the intake of plant-based ingredients per meal to feel fuller and less prone to satisfy a craving. Throughout the fourth week of the program and after, you are going to be learning about new recipes that involve great plant-based meals. Learning new recipes is going to help you keep your meal plan diverse and full of nutrients. Your plant-based diet adventure does not end with this program! After the fourth week, you will be used to this type of diet but you will still have a lot to learn and a lot of material to experiment with. One very important thing to learn at this stage of the program is that you should be eating plant based, healthy snacks every day to feel fuller and reduce cravings, as well as stay energetic and productive throughout the day. Stay consistent with your meal plans and include snacks every now and then. Of course, the easiest and always go to snack should be fruit and vegetables or nuts. There is nothing easier than pull out an apple or few nuts from your bag when on the go. To make your transition smoother, make always sure you have a little snack always with you, so you don't end up eating fast food or some other processed foods. Remember you came to this world with only one body and you are not getting any other. So, you better take good care of it.

Did you have fun in the kitchen last three weeks and you feel like discovering more fun recipes, that can make your snacks more diverse and creative? Here are three great recipes for plant-based snacks!

#1 Two-Ingredients Banana- Oatmeal cookies

Ingredients:

1 large ripe banana

1 cup oats

Directions:

Simply mash the banana and mix in the oats. If desired you can still add one of following ingredients (raisins, dried cranberries, cocoa nibs, shredded coconut, chopped nuts).

Shape tablespoons of dough on a baking sheet in a form of cookies.  Bake in the oven heated on 180°C for about 10 minutes. Let them cool after taking out of the oven and enjoy.

#2 Coconut Bites

Ingredients:

1 cup of pineapple juice

2 cups of diced mango

2 diced ripe bananas

½ vanilla bean

4 cups of shredded coconut

¾ cup of toasted shredded coconut

Directions:

Use a small pot to cook the pineapple juice, bananas, mango and vanilla. Cook at low heat for five minutes. Then scrape the seeds from the vanilla bean into the pot and cook for two more minutes. Put the ingredients into the pot, process the 4 cups of shredded coconut until you have a smooth but firm mixture. Let the mixture cool down for an hour or two and then a roll small amount of it into a ball and roll it into the toasted coconut. Roll up all your coconut bites for a perfect plant-based snack!

#3 Fruit Pie

Ingredients:

1 cup of pitted dates

1 ½ cup of walnuts or pecans

1 tablespoon of vanilla extract

½ cup of shredded coconut

½ tablespoon of cinnamon

Sliced fresh fruit

Directions:

Put all crust ingredients into a food processor and blend them until you get a paste. Press the paste into a pie pan and let it chill for a while, until it is ready to add fruit on it. Arrange the fruit on top of the pie according to your liking and cool the pie off 1 hour before serving and, voila, a perfect, healthy snack.

This plant-based diet guide was designed to introduce beginners to this kind of diet and encourage them to make the right choices regarding their eating habits. As a beginner, you don't have to feel overwhelmed and pressured by diet plans. Instead of jumping straight into it, it is more important to firstly get to know the diet and learn why it is beneficial for your health and overall well-being.  That's exactly what this book was designed to do, teach you about the plant-based diet and show you how to gradually yet surly transition to a diet without any animal products. What you should take away from this book are all the reasons why the plant-based diet positively affects your health and why it is important to manage your eating habits regularly. Upon getting to know all this information, the next step is to start implementing it in your everyday life. Ditching animal products completely sounds like a difficult task but it can actually be easy and effortless, as long as you follow the right meal plan. My plant-based diet guide will help you effortlessly transition to a plant-based diet by introducing new ingredients gradually, without pressure. Throughout this 4-week program, you will get used to plant-based ingredients and start letting go of animal products up until the point where you completely throw them out of your everyday meals.  Keep in mind that diet transition is a steady process, so don't try to rush and skip steps of the meal program in hopes to achieve the results sooner. Take it easy and enjoy combining various delicious ingredients and preparing outstanding meals while receiving all the necessary nutrients for your body's proper functioning.

# Chapter 6 The Recipes

**Breakfast**

**Fruity Granola**

Preparation Time: 15 Minutes

Cooking Time: 45 Minutes

Servings: 5

**Ingredients**

2 cups rolled oats

¾ cup whole-wheat flour

1 tablespoon ground cinnamon

1 teaspoon ground ginger (optional)

½ cup sunflower seeds, or walnuts, chopped

½ cup almonds, chopped

½ cup pumpkin seeds

½ cup unsweetened shredded coconut

1¼ cups pure fruit juice (cranberry, apple, or something similar)

½ cup raisins, or dried cranberries

½ cup goji berries (optional)

**Directions**

Preheat the oven to 350°F.

Mix together the oats, flour, cinnamon, ginger, sunflower seeds, almonds, pumpkin seeds, and coconut in a large bowl.

Sprinkle the juice over the mixture, and stir until it's just moistened. You might need a bit more or a bit less liquid, depending on how much your oats and flour absorb.

Spread the granola on a large baking sheet (the more spread out it is the better), and put it in the oven. After about 15 minutes, use a spatula to turn the granola so that the middle gets dried out. Let the granola bake until it's as crunchy as you want it, about 30 minutes more.

Take the granola out of the oven and stir in the raisins and goji berries (if using). Store leftovers in an airtight container for up to 2 weeks.

Serve with non-dairy milk and fresh fruit, use as a topper for morning porridge or a smoothie bowl to add a bit of crunch, or make a granola parfait by layering with non-dairy yogurt or puréed banana.

Per Serving (½ cup) Calories: 398; Protein: 11g; Total fat: 25g; Carbohydrates: 39g; Fiber: 8g

**Pumpkin Steel-Cut Oats**
Preparation Time: 2 Minutes

Cooking Time: 35 Minutes

Servings: 4

**Ingredients**

3 cups water

1 cup steel-cut oats

½ cup canned pumpkin purée

¼ cup pumpkin seeds (pepitas)

2 tablespoons maple syrup

Pinch salt

**Directions**

In a large saucepan, bring the water to a boil.

Add the oats, stir, and reduce the heat to low. Simmer until the oats are soft, 20 to 30 minutes, continuing to stir occasionally.

Stir in the pumpkin purée and continue cooking on low for 3 to 5 minutes longer. Stir in the pumpkin seeds and maple syrup, and season with the salt.

Divide the oatmeal into 4 single-serving containers. Let cool before sealing the lids.

Place the airtight containers in the refrigerator for 5 days or freeze for up to 3 months. To thaw, refrigerate overnight. Reheat in the microwave for 2½ minutes or in a skillet over medium-high heat for 6 to 8 minutes.

Nutrition: Calories:121; Protein: 4g; Total fat: 5g; Carbohydrates: 17g; Fiber: 2g

**Granola**

PREPARATION TIME: 5 MINUTES

Cooking Time: 15 MINUTES

Servings: about 8 cups

**Ingredients**

51/2 cups old-fashioned oats

11/2 cups slivered almonds

1/2 cup shelled sunflower seeds

1 cup golden raisins

1 cup shredded unsweetened coconut

1 cup pure maple syrup

1/2 teaspoon ground cinnamon

1/4 teaspoon ground allspice

Pinch salt

**Directions**

Preheat the oven to 325°F. Spread the oats, almonds, and sunflower seeds in a 9 x 13-inch baking pan and place in the oven for 10 minutes.

Remove from the oven and reduce the temperature to 300°F. Add the raisins, coconut, maple syrup, cinnamon, allspice, and salt and stir to combine.

Return the pan to the oven and bake for 15 minutes, or until the mixture is crisp and dry. Be careful not to burn.

Remove from oven and let cool completely, 30 minutes. Transfer to an airtight container and store in the refrigerator where it will keep for several weeks.

## Chocolate Quinoa Breakfast Bowl

Preparation Time: 5 Minutes

Cooking Time: 30 Minutes

Servings: 2

**Ingredients**

1 cup quinoa

1 teaspoon ground cinnamon

1 cup non-dairy milk

1 cup water

1 large banana

2 to 3 tablespoons unsweetened cocoa powder, or carob

1 to 2 tablespoons almond butter, or other nut or seed butter

1 tablespoon ground flaxseed, or chia or hemp seeds

2 tablespoons walnuts

¼ cup raspberries

**Directions**

Put the quinoa, cinnamon, milk, and water in a medium pot. Bring to a boil over high heat, then turn down low and simmer, covered, for 25 to 30 minutes.

While the quinoa is simmering, purée or mash the banana in a medium bowl and stir in the cocoa powder, almond butter, and flaxseed.

To serve, spoon 1 cup cooked quinoa into a bowl, top with half the pudding and half the walnuts and raspberries.

Nutrition: Calories: 392; Protein: 12g; Total fat: 19g; Saturated fat: 1g; Carbohydrates: 49g; Fiber: 10g

**Savory Oatmeal Porridge**
Preparation Time: 2 Minutes

Cooking Time: 25 Minutes

Servings: 4

**Ingredients**

2½ cups vegetable broth

2½ cups unsweetened almond milk or other plant-based milk

½ cup steel-cut oats

1 tablespoon farro

½ cup slivered almonds

¼ cup nutritional yeast

2 cups old-fashioned rolled oats

½ teaspoon salt (optional)

**Directions**

In a large saucepan or pot, bring the broth and almond milk to a boil. Add the oats, farro, almond slivers, and nutritional yeast. Cook over medium-high heat for 20 minutes, stirring occasionally.

Add the rolled oats and cook for another 5 minutes, until creamy. Stir in the salt (if using).

Divide into 4 single-serving containers.

Let cool before sealing the lids. Place the airtight containers in the refrigerator for 5 days or freeze for up to 3 months. To thaw, refrigerate overnight. Reheat in the microwave for 2½ minutes or in a skillet over medium-high heat for 6 to 8 minutes.

Nutrition: Calories: 208; Protein: 14g; Total fat: 8g; Saturated fat: 1g; Carbohydrates: 22g; Fiber: 7g

**Muesli and Berries Bowl**
Preparation Time: 10 Minutes

Cooking Time: 0 Minutes

Servings: 5

**Ingredients**

**FOR THE MUESLI**

1 cup rolled oats

1 cup spelt flakes, or quinoa flakes, or more rolled oats

2 cups puffed cereal

¼ cup sunflower seeds

¼ cup almonds

¼ cup raisins

¼ cup dried cranberries

¼ cup chopped dried figs

¼ cup unsweetened shredded coconut

¼ cup non-dairy chocolate chips

1 to 3 teaspoons ground cinnamon

**FOR THE BOWL**

½ cup non-dairy milk, or unsweetened applesauce

¾ cup muesli

½ cup berries

**Directions**

Put the muesli ingredients in a container or bag and shake.

Combine the muesli and bowl ingredients in a bowl or to-go container.

Substitutions: Try chopped Brazil nuts, peanuts, dried cranberries, dried blueberries, dried mango, or whatever inspires you. Ginger and cardamom are interesting flavors if you want to branch out on spices.

Nutrition: Calories: 441; Protein: 10g; Total fat: 20g; Carbohydrates: 63g; Fiber: 13g

**Breakfast Casserole**
Preparation Time: 15 Minutes

Cooking Time: 0 Minutes

Servings: 6 Servings

**Ingredients**

1 cup quick-cooking grits

1/2 cup shredded vegan Cheddar cheese

2 tablespoons vegan margarine

1 cup cooked and chopped tempeh bacon or vegan sausage

1 cup fresh or frozen corn kernels

**Directions**

Preheat the oven to 375°F. Lightly oil a 9 x 13-inch baking pan and set aside.

In a large saucepan, combine the soy milk and broth and bring to a boil over high heat. Add salt to taste (depending on the saltiness of your broth) and stir in the grits. Reduce the heat to low and cook, stirring occasionally, until the grits are thickened but not stiff. Turn off the heat and stir in the cheese, margarine, tempeh bacon, and corn.

Scrape the mixture into the prepared baking pan. Spread evenly, smooth the top, and bake until slightly puffed and golden brown, about 45 minutes. Serve immediately.

**Cinnamon And Spice Overnight Oats**

PREPARATION TIME: 10 MINUTES • OVERNIGHT TO SOAK

Servings: 5

**Ingredients**

2½ cups old-fashioned rolled oats

5 tablespoons pumpkin seeds (pepitas)

5 tablespoons chopped pecans

5 cups unsweetened plant-based milk

2½ teaspoons maple syrup or agave syrup

½ to 1 teaspoon salt

½ to 1 teaspoon ground cinnamon

½ to 1 teaspoon ground ginger

Fresh fruit (optional)

**Directions**

Line up 5 wide-mouth pint jars. In each jar, combine ½ cup of oats, 1 tablespoon of pumpkin seeds, 1 tablespoon of pecans, 1 cup of plant-based milk, ½ teaspoon of maple syrup, 1 pinch of salt, 1 pinch of cinnamon, and 1 pinch of ginger.

Stir the ingredients in each jar. Close the jars tightly with lids. To serve, top with fresh fruit (if using). Place the airtight jars in the refrigerator at least overnight before eating and for up to 5 days.

Nutrition: Calories:177; Protein: 6g; Total fat: 9g; Carbohydrates: 19g; Fiber: 4g

## Baked Banana French Toast with Raspberry Syrup

Preparation Time: 10 Minutes

Cooking Time: 30 Minutes

Servings: 8 Slices

**Ingredients**

**FOR THE FRENCH TOAST**

1 banana

1 cup coconut milk

1 teaspoon pure vanilla extract

¼ teaspoon ground nutmeg

½ teaspoon ground cinnamon

1½ teaspoons arrowroot powder

Pinch sea salt

8 slices whole-grain bread

FOR THE RASPBERRY SYRUP

1 cup fresh or frozen raspberries, or other berries

2 tablespoons water, or pure fruit juice

1 to 2 tablespoons maple syrup, or coconut sugar (optional)

**Directions**

Preheat the oven to 350°F.

In a shallow bowl, purée or mash the banana well. Mix in the coconut milk, vanilla, nutmeg, cinnamon, arrowroot, and salt.

Dip the slices of bread in the banana mixture, and then lay them out in a 13-by-9-inch baking dish. They should cover the bottom of the dish and can overlap a bit but shouldn't be stacked on top of each other. Pour any leftover banana mixture over the bread, and put the dish in the oven.

Bake about 30 minutes, or until the tops are lightly browned.

Serve topped with raspberry syrup.

To Make the Raspberry Syrup

Heat the raspberries in a small pot with the water and the maple syrup (if using) on medium heat.

Leave to simmer, stirring occasionally and breaking up the berries, for 15 to 20 minutes, until the liquid has reduced.

Leftover raspberry syrup makes a great topping for simple oatmeal as a quick and delicious breakfast, or as a drizzle on top of whole-grain toast smeared with natural peanut butter.

Nutrition: Calories: 166; Protein: 5g; Total fat: 7g; Saturated fat: 1g; Carbohydrates: 23g;

**Great Green Smoothie**
Preparation Time: 5 Minutes

Cooking Time: 0 Minutes

Servings: 4

**Ingredients**

4 bananas, peeled

4 cups hulled strawberries

4 cups spinach

4 cups plant-based milk

**Directions**

Open 4 quart-size, freezer-safe bags. In each, layer in the following order: 1 banana (halved or sliced), 1 cup of strawberries, and 1 cup of spinach. Seal and place in the freezer.

To serve, take a frozen bag of Great Green Smoothie ingredients and transfer to a blender. Add 1 cup of plant-based milk, and blend until smooth. Place freezer bags in the freezer for up to 2 months.

Nutrition: Calories: 173; Protein: 4g; Total fat: 2g; Carbohydrates: 40g; Fiber: 7g

**Breakfast Bulgur With Pears And Pecans**
Preparation Time: 5 Minutes

Cooking Time: 15 Minutes

Servings: 4 Servings

**Ingredients**

2 cups water

1/2 teaspoon salt

1 cup medium bulgur

1 tablespoon vegan margarine

2 ripe pears, peeled, cored, and chopped

1/4 cup chopped pecans

**Directions**

In a large saucepan, bring the water to a boil over high heat. Add the salt and stir in the bulgur. Reduce heat to low, cover, and simmer until the bulgur is tender and liquid has absorbed, about 15 minutes.

Remove from the heat and stir in the margarine, pears, and pecans. Cover and let sit for 12 to 15 minutes more before serving.

**Sunshine Muffins**

PREPARATION TIME: 15 MINUTES

Cooking Time: 30 MINUTES

Servings: 6

**Ingredients**

1 teaspoon coconut oil, for greasing muffin tins (optional)

2 tablespoons almond butter, or sunflower seed butter

¼ cup non-dairy milk

1 orange, peeled

1 carrot, coarsely chopped

2 tablespoons chopped dried apricots, or other dried fruit

3 tablespoons molasses

2 tablespoons ground flaxseed

1 teaspoon apple cider vinegar

1 teaspoon pure vanilla extract

½ teaspoon ground cinnamon

½ teaspoon ground ginger (optional)

¼ teaspoon ground nutmeg (optional)

¼ teaspoon allspice (optional)

¾ cup rolled oats, or whole-wheat flour

1 teaspoon baking powder

½ teaspoon baking soda

MIX-INS (OPTIONAL)

½ cup rolled oats

2 tablespoons raisins, or other chopped dried fruit

2 tablespoons sunflower seeds

**Directions**

Preheat the oven to 350°F.

Prepare a 6-cup muffin tin by rubbing the insides of the cups with coconut oil or using silicone or paper muffin cups.

Purée the nut butter, milk, orange, carrot, apricots, molasses, flaxseed, vinegar, vanilla, cinnamon, ginger, nutmeg, and allspice in a food processor or blender until somewhat smooth.

Grind the oats in a clean coffee grinder until they're the consistency of flour (or use whole-grain flour). In a large bowl, mix the oats with the baking powder and baking soda. Mix the wet ingredients into the dry ingredients until just combined. Fold in the mix-ins (if using). Spoon about ¼ cup batter into each muffin cup and bake for 30 minutes, or until a toothpick inserted into the center comes out clean.

The orange creates a very moist base, so the muffins may take longer than 30 minutes, depending on how heavy your muffin tin is. Store the muffins in the fridge or freezer, because they are so moist. If you plan to keep them frozen, you can easily double the batch for a full dozen.

Nutrition: Calories: 287; Protein: 8g; Total fat: 12g; Carbohydrates: 41g; Fiber: 6g

**Breakfast Bran Muffins**
Preparation Time: 10 Minutes

Cooking Time: 20 Minutes

Servings: 12 Muffins

**Ingredients**

3 cups bran flakes cereal

11/2 cups. Whole-wheat flour

1/2 cup raisins

3 teaspoons baking powder

1/2 teaspoon ground cinnamon

1/2 teaspoon salt

1/3 cup brown sugar

¾ cup fresh orange juice

**Directions**

Preheat the oven to 400°F. Lightly oil a 12-cup muffin tin or line it with paper liners and set aside.

In a large bowl, combine the bran flakes, flour, raisins, baking powder, cinnamon, and salt.

In a medium bowl, combine the sugar, orange juice, and oil and mix until blended. Pour the wet Ingredients into the dry Ingredients and mix until just moistened.

Fill the cups about two-thirds full. Bake until golden brown and a toothpick inserted into a muffin comes out clean, about 20 minutes. Serve warm.

**Smoothie Breakfast Bowl**
PREPARATION TIME: 10 MINUTES

Cooking Time: 0 MINUTES

Servings: 4

**Ingredients**

4 bananas, peeled

1 cup dragon fruit or fruit of choice

1 cup Baked Granola

2 cups fresh berries

½ cup slivered almonds

4 cups plant-based milk

**Directions**

Open 4 quart-size, freezer-safe bags, and layer in the following order: 1 banana (halved or sliced) and ¼ cup dragon fruit. Into 4 small jelly jars, layer in the following order: ¼ cup granola, ½ cup berries, and 2 tablespoons slivered almonds.

To serve, take a frozen bag of bananas and dragon fruit and transfer to a blender. Add 1 cup of plant-based milk, and blend until smooth. Pour into a bowl. Add the contents of 1 jar of granola, berries, and almonds over the top of the smoothie, and serve with a spoon. Place the freezer bags in the freezer for up to 2 months. Store the jars of berries, granola, and nuts in the refrigerator for up to 1 week.

Nutrition: Calories: 384; Protein: 6g; Total fat: 5g; Carbohydrates: 57g; Fiber: 8g

**Pink Panther Smoothie**
PREPARATION TIME: 5 MINUTES

Cooking Time: 0 MINUTES

Servings: 3 CUPS

**Ingredients**

1 cup strawberries

1 cup chopped melon (any kind)

1 cup cranberries, or raspberries

1 tablespoon chia seeds

½ cup coconut milk, or other non-dairy milk

1 cup water

(OPTIONAL)

1 teaspoon goji berries

2 tablespoons fresh mint, chopped

**Directions**

Purée everything in a blender until smooth, adding more water (or coconut milk) if needed.

Add bonus boosters, as desired. Purée until blended. If you don't have (or don't like) coconut, try using sunflower seeds for an immune boost of zinc and selenium.

Per Serving 3 Cups: Calories: 459; Protein: 8g; Total fat: 30g; Carbohydrates: 52g; Fiber: 19g

**Mango Madness**
PREPARATION TIME: 5 MINUTES

Cooking Time: 0 MINUTES

Servings: 4 CUPS

**Ingredients**

1 banana

1 cup chopped mango (frozen or fresh)

1 cup chopped peach (frozen or fresh)

1 cup strawberries

1 carrot, peeled and chopped (optional)

1 cup water

**Directions**

Purée everything in a blender until smooth, adding more water if needed.

If you can't find frozen peaches and fresh ones aren't in season, just use extra mango or strawberries, or try cantaloupe.

Nutrition: Calories: 376; Protein: 5g; Total fat: 2g; Carbohydrates: 95g; Fiber: 14g

**Savory Pancakes**

Preparation Time: 10 Minutes

Cooking Time: 15 Minutes

Servings: 4

**Ingredients**

1 cup whole-wheat flour

1 teaspoon garlic salt

1 teaspoon onion powder

½ teaspoon baking soda

¼ teaspoon salt

1 cup lightly pressed, crumbled soft or firm tofu

⅓ cup unsweetened plant-based milk

¼ cup lemon juice (about 2 small lemons)

2 tablespoons extra-virgin olive oil

½ cup finely chopped mushrooms

½ cup finely chopped onion

2 cups tightly packed greens (arugula, spinach, or baby kale work great)

Nonstick cooking spray

**Directions**

In a large bowl, combine the flour, garlic salt, onion powder, baking soda, and salt. Mix well. In a blender, combine the tofu, plant-based milk, lemon juice, and olive oil. Purée on high speed for 30 seconds.

Pour the contents of the blender into the bowl of dry ingredients and whisk until combined well. Fold in the mushrooms, onion, and greens.

Spray a large skillet or griddle pan with nonstick cooking spray and set over medium-high heat. Reduce the heat to medium and add ½ cup of batter per pancake. Cook on both sides for about 3 minutes, or until set. After flipping, press down on the cooked side of the pancake with a spatula to flatten out the pancake. Repeat until the batter is gone.

Divide the cooked pancakes among 4 single-serving containers. Let cool before sealing the lids.

Place the airtight storage containers in the refrigerator for up to 4 days. To reheat, microwave for 1½ to 2 minutes. To freeze, place the pancakes on a parchment paper–lined baking sheet in a single layer. If there's more than one layer, place another piece of parchment paper over the pancakes and place the second layer on top. Place the baking sheet in the freezer for 2 to 4 hours. Transfer the frozen pancakes to a freezer-safe bag (cut the parchment paper and place a small piece between each pancake). To thaw, refrigerate overnight. Preheat an oven or toaster oven to 350ºF. Place the pancakes on a parchment paper–lined baking sheet and bake for 10 to 15 minutes, or stack the pancakes on a plate and microwave for 2 to 3 minutes.

Nutrition: Calories: 246; Protein: 10g; Total fat: 11g; Carbohydrates: 30g; Fiber: 3g

**Maple-Pecan Waffles**

Preparation Time: 10 Minutes

Cooking Time: 5 Minutes

Servings: 4 Servings

**Ingredients**

1¾ cups whole-wheat flour

1/3 cup coarsely ground pecans

1 tablespoon baking powder

1/2 teaspoon salt

11/2 cups soy milk

3 tablespoons pure maple syrup

3 tablespoons vegan margarine, melted

**Directions**

Lightly oil the waffle iron and preheat it. Preheat the oven to 225°F.

In a large bowl, combine the flour, pecans, baking powder, and salt. Set aside.

In a medium bowl, whisk together the soy milk, maple syrup, and margarine. Add the wet Ingredients to the dry

Ingredients and blend with a few swift strokes, mixing until just combined.

Ladle 1/2 to 1 cup of the batter (depending on the Directions with your waffle iron) onto the hot waffle iron. Cook until done, 3 to 5 minutes for most waffle irons. Transfer the cooked waffles to a heatproof platter and keep warm in the oven while cooking the rest of the waffles.

## Lemon-Kissed Blueberry Waffles

Preparation Time: 10 Minutes

Cooking Time: 5 Minutes

Servings: 4 Servings

## Ingredients

11/2 cups whole-heat flour

1/2 cup old-fashioned oats

1/4 cup sugar

3 teaspoons baking powder

1/2 teaspoon salt

1 teaspoon ground cinnamon

2 cups soy milk

1 tablespoon fresh lemon juice

1 teaspoon lemon zest

1/4 cup vegan margarine, melted

1/2 cup fresh blueberries

## Directions

Lightly oil the waffle iron and preheat it. Preheat the oven to 225°F.

In a large bowl, combine the flour, oats, sugar, baking powder, salt, and cinnamon. Set aside.

In a separate large bowl, whisk together the soy milk, lemon juice, lemon zest, and margarine. Add the wet Ingredients to the dry Ingredients and blend with a few swift strokes, mixing until just combined. Fold in the blueberries.

Ladle 1/2 to 1 cup of the batter (depending on the Directions with your waffle iron) onto the hot waffle iron. Cook until done, 3 to 5 minutes for most waffle irons. Transfer the cooked waffles to a heatproof platter and keep warm in the oven while cooking the rest.

## Tropi-Kale Breeze
Preparation Time: 5 Minutes

Cooking Time: 0minutes

Servings: 4

## Ingredients

1 cup chopped pineapple (frozen or fresh)

1 cup chopped mango (frozen or fresh)

½ to 1 cup chopped kale

½ avocado

½ cup coconut milk

1 cup water, or coconut water

1 teaspoon matcha green tea powder (optional)

**Directions**

Purée everything in a blender until smooth, adding more water (or coconut milk) if needed.

Nutrition: Calories: 566; Protein: 8g; Total fat: 36g; Saturated fat: 1g; Carbohydrates: 66g; Fiber: 12g

**Tofu-Spinach Scramble**
Preparation Time: 20 Minutes

Cooking Time: 15 Minutes

Servings: 5

**Ingredients**

1 (14-ounce) package water-packed extra-firm tofu

1 teaspoon extra-virgin olive oil or ¼ cup vegetable broth

1 small yellow onion, diced

3 teaspoons minced garlic (about 3 cloves)

3 large celery stalks, chopped

2 large carrots, peeled (optional) and chopped

1 teaspoon chili powder

½ teaspoon ground cumin

½ teaspoon ground turmeric

½ teaspoon salt (optional)

¼ teaspoon freshly ground black pepper

5 cups loosely packed spinach

**Directions**

Press and drain the tofu by placing it, wrapped in a paper towel, on a plate in the sink. Place a cutting board over the tofu, then set a heavy pot, can, or cookbook on the cutting board. Remove after 10 minutes. (Alternatively, use a tofu press.)

In a medium bowl, crumble the tofu with your hands or a potato masher. Set aside.

In a large skillet over medium-high heat, heat the olive oil. Add the onion, garlic, celery, and carrots, and sauté for 5 minutes, until the onion is softened.

Add the crumbled tofu, chili powder, cumin, turmeric, salt (if using), and pepper, and continue cooking for 7 to 8 more minutes, stirring frequently, until the tofu begins to brown.

Add the spinach and mix well. Cover and reduce the heat to medium. Steam the spinach for 3 minutes.

Divide evenly among 5 single-serving containers. Let cool before sealing the lids.

Place the airtight containers in the refrigerator for 5 days or freeze for up to 1 month. To thaw, refrigerate overnight. Reheat in the microwave for 2½ minutes or in a skillet over medium-high heat for 6 to 8 minutes.

Nutrition: Calories: 170; Protein: 7g; Total fat: 9g; Carbohydrates: 9g; Fiber: 3g

**Chai Chia Smoothie**
Preparation Time: 5 Minutes

Cooking Time: 0minutes

Servings: 3

**Ingredients**

1 banana

½ cup coconut milk

1 cup water

1 cup alfalfa sprouts (optional)

1 to 2 soft Medjool dates, pitted

1 tablespoon chia seeds, or ground flax or hemp hearts

¼ teaspoon ground cinnamon

Pinch ground cardamom

1 tablespoon grated fresh ginger, or ¼ teaspoon ground ginger

**Directions**

Purée everything in a blender until smooth, adding more water (or coconut milk) if needed.

Although dates are super sweet, they don't cause a large blood sugar spike. They're great to boost sweetness while also boosting your intake of fiber and potassium. Per Serving (3 cups)

Nutrition: Calories: 477; Protein: 7g; Total fat: 29g; Carbohydrates: 57g; Fiber: 14g

## Broiled Grapefruit with Cinnamon Pitas

Preparation Time: 10 Minutes

Cooking Time: 15 Minutes

Servings: 5

### Ingredients

2 whole-wheat pitas, cut into wedges

2 tablespoons coconut oil, melted

1 tablespoon ground cinnamon

2 tablespoons brown sugar

1 grapefruit, halved

2 tablespoons pure maple syrup or agave

### Directions

Preheat the oven to 375°F.

Line a baking sheet with parchment paper.

Spread pita wedges in a single layer on a baking sheet and brush with melted coconut oil.

In a small bowl, combine the cinnamon and brown sugar and sprinkle over the pita wedges.

Bake in preheated oven until the wedges are crisp, about 8 minutes. Transfer the pita wedges to a plate and set aside.

Turn the oven to broil. Place the grapefruit halves on the baking sheet. Drizzle the maple syrup over the top of the grapefruit, if using. Broil until the syrup bubbles and begins to crystallize, 3 to 5 minutes. Serve immediately.

**Blueberry Oatmeal Breakfast Bars**
Preparation Time: 10 Minutes

Cooking Time: 40 Minutes

Servings: 12

**Ingredients**

2 cups uncooked rolled oats

2 cups all-purpose flour

1½ cups dark-brown sugar

1½ teaspoons baking soda

½ teaspoon sea salt

½ teaspoon ground cinnamon

1 cup vegan butter, melted

4 cups blueberries, fresh or frozen

¼ cup organic cane sugar

2 tablespoons cornstarch

**Directions**

Preheat the oven to 375°F. Lightly grease a 9-by-13-inch baking dish.

In a large bowl, combine the oats, flour, sugar, baking soda, salt, and cinnamon. Add the butter and mix until well incorporated and crumbly.

In a separate large bowl, combine the blueberries, cane sugar, and cornstarch, mixing until the blueberries are evenly coated.

Press 3 cups of the oatmeal mixture into the prepared baking pan. Spread the blueberry mixture on top and crumble the remaining oatmeal mixture over the blueberries.

Bake for 40 minutes.

Remove from the oven and let cool completely before cutting into bars.

## Chocolate PB Smoothie
Preparation Time: 5 Minutes

Cooking Time: 0 Minutes

Servings: 4

### Ingredients

1 banana

¼ cup rolled oats, or 1 scoop plant protein powder

1 tablespoon flaxseed, or chia seeds

1 tablespoon unsweetened cocoa powder

1 tablespoon peanut butter, or almond or sunflower seed butter

1 tablespoon maple syrup (optional)

1 cup alfalfa sprouts, or spinach, chopped (optional)

½ cup non-dairy milk (optional)

1 cup water

**OPTIONAL**

1 teaspoon maca powder

1 teaspoon cocoa nibs

**Directions**

Purée everything in a blender until smooth, adding more water (or non-dairy milk) if needed. Add bonus boosters, as desired. Purée until blended.

Nutrition: Calories: 474; Protein: 13g; Total fat: 16g; Carbohydrates: 79g; Fiber: 18g

# Lunch

## Cashew Siam Salad

Preparation Time: 10 minutes

Cooking Time: 3 minutes

Servings: 4

**Ingredients:**

Salad:

4 cups baby spinach, rinsed, drained

½ cup pickled red cabbage

Dressing:

1-inch piece ginger, finely chopped

1 tsp. chili garlic paste

1 tbsp. soy sauce

½ tbsp. rice vinegar

1 tbsp. sesame oil

3 tbsp. avocado oil

Toppings:

½ cup raw cashews, unsalted

¼ cup fresh cilantro, chopped

**Directions:**

Put the spinach and red cabbage in a large bowl. Toss to combine and set the salad aside.

Toast the cashews in a frying pan over medium-high heat, stirring occasionally until the cashews are golden brown. This should take about 3 minutes. Turn off the heat and set the frying pan aside.

Mix all the dressing ingredients in a medium-sized bowl and use a spoon to mix them into a smooth dressing.

Pour the dressing over the spinach salad and top with the toasted cashews.

Toss the salad to combine all ingredients and transfer the large bowl to the fridge. Allow the salad to chill for up to one hour – doing so will guarantee a better flavor. Alternatively, the salad can be served right away, topped with the optional cilantro. Enjoy!

Nutrition:

Calories 236

Carbohydrates 6.1 g

Fats 21.6 g

Protein 4.2 g

**Avocado and Cauliflower Hummus**
Preparation Time: 5 minutes

Cooking Time: 25 minutes

Servings: 2

**Ingredients:**
1 medium cauliflower, stem removed and chopped
1 large Hass avocado, peeled, pitted, and chopped

¼ cup extra virgin olive oil

2 garlic cloves

½ tbsp. lemon juice

½ tsp. onion powder

Sea salt and ground black pepper to taste

2 large carrots

¼ cup fresh cilantro, chopped

**Directions:**

Preheat the oven to 450°F, and line a baking tray with aluminum foil.

Put the chopped cauliflower on the baking tray and drizzle with 2 tablespoons of olive oil.

Roast the chopped cauliflower in the oven for 20-25 minutes, until lightly brown.

Remove the tray from the oven and allow the cauliflower to cool down.

Add all the ingredients—except the carrots and optional fresh cilantro—to a food processor or blender, and blend the ingredients into a smooth hummus.

Transfer the hummus to a medium-sized bowl, cover, and put it in the fridge for at least 30 minutes.

Take the hummus out of the fridge and, if desired, top it with the optional chopped cilantro and more salt and pepper to taste; serve with the carrot fries, and enjoy!

Nutrition:

Calories 416

Carbohydrates 8.4 g

Fats 40.3 g

Protein 3.3 g

**Raw Zoodles with Avocado 'N Nuts**
Preparation Time: 10 minutes

Servings: 2

**Ingredients:**

1 medium zucchini

1½ cups basil

1/3 cup water

5 tbsp. pine nuts

2 tbsp. lemon juice

1 medium avocado, peeled, pitted, sliced

Optional: 2 tbsp. olive oil

6 yellow cherry tomatoes, halved

Optional: 6 red cherry tomatoes, halved

Sea salt and black pepper to taste

**Directions:**

Add the basil, water, nuts, lemon juice, avocado slices, optional olive oil (if desired), salt, and pepper to a blender.

Blend the ingredients into a smooth mixture. Add more salt and pepper to taste and blend again.

Divide the sauce and the zucchini noodles between two medium-sized bowls for serving, and combine in each.

Top the mixtures with the halved yellow cherry tomatoes, and the optional red cherry tomatoes (if desired); serve and enjoy!

Nutrition:

Calories 317

Carbohydrates 7.4 g

Fats 28.1 g

Protein 7.2 g

**Cauliflower Sushi**
Preparation Time: 30 minutes

Servings: 4

**Ingredients:**

Sushi Base:

6 cups cauliflower florets

½ cup vegan cheese

1 medium spring onion, diced

4 nori sheets

Sea salt and pepper to taste

1 tbsp. rice vinegar or sushi vinegar

1 medium garlic clove, minced

Filling:

1 medium Hass avocado, peeled, sliced

½ medium cucumber, skinned, sliced

4 asparagus spears

A handful of enoki mushrooms

**Directions:**

Put the cauliflower florets in a food processor or blender. Pulse the florets into a rice-like substance. When using readymade cauliflower rice, add this to the blender.

Add the vegan cheese, spring onions, and vinegar to the food processor or blender. Top these ingredients with salt and pepper to taste, and pulse everything into a chunky mixture. Make sure not to turn the ingredients into a puree by pulsing too long.

Taste and add more vinegar, salt, or pepper to taste. Add the optional minced garlic clove to the blender and pulse again for a few seconds.

Lay out the nori sheets and spread the cauliflower rice mixture out evenly between the sheets. Make sure to leave at least 2 inches of the top and bottom edges empty.

Place one or more combinations of multiple filling ingredients along the center of the spread out rice mixture. Experiment with different ingredients per nori sheet for the best flavor.

Roll up each nori sheet tightly. (Using a sushi mat will make this easier.)

Either serve the sushi as a nori roll, or, slice each roll up into sushi pieces.

Serve right away with a small amount of wasabi, pickled ginger, and soy sauce!

Nutrition:

Calories 189

Carbohydrates 7.6 g

Fats 14.4 g

Protein 6.1 g

**Spinach and Mashed Tofu Salad**
Preparation Time: 20 minutes

Servings: 4

**Ingredients:**

2 8-oz. blocks firm tofu, drained

4 cups baby spinach leaves

4 tbsp. cashew butter

1½ tbsp. soy sauce

1-inch piece ginger, finely chopped

1 tsp. red miso paste

2 tbsp. sesame seeds

1 tsp. organic orange zest

1 tsp. nori flakes

2 tbsp. water

**Directions:**

Use paper towels to absorb any excess water left in the tofu before crumbling both blocks into small pieces.

In a large bowl, combine the mashed tofu with the spinach leaves.

Mix the remaining ingredients in another small bowl and, if desired, add the optional water for a smoother dressing.

Pour this dressing over the mashed tofu and spinach leaves.

Transfer the bowl to the fridge and allow the salad to chill for up to one hour. Doing so will guarantee a better flavor. Or, the salad can be served right away. Enjoy!

Nutrition:

Calories 166

Carbohydrates 5.5 g

Fats 10.7 g

Protein 11.3 g

**Cucumber Edamame Salad**
Preparation Time: 5 minutes

Cooking Time: 8 minutes

Servings: 2

**Ingredients:**

3 tbsp. avocado oil

1 cup cucumber, sliced into thin rounds

½ cup fresh sugar snap peas, sliced or whole

½ cup fresh edamame

¼ cup radish, sliced

1 large Hass avocado, peeled, pitted, sliced

1 nori sheet, crumbled

2 tsp. roasted sesame seeds

1 tsp. salt

**Directions:**

Bring a medium-sized pot filled halfway with water to a boil over medium-high heat.

Add the sugar snaps and cook them for about 2 minutes.

Take the pot off the heat, drain the excess water, transfer the sugar snaps to a medium-sized bowl and set aside for now.

Fill the pot with water again, add the teaspoon of salt and bring to a boil over medium-high heat.

Add the edamame to the pot and let them cook for about 6 minutes.

Take the pot off the heat, drain the excess water, transfer the soybeans to the bowl with sugar snaps and let them cool down for about 5 minutes.

Combine all ingredients, except the nori crumbs and roasted sesame seeds, in a medium-sized bowl.

Carefully stir, using a spoon, until all ingredients are evenly coated in oil.

Top the salad with the nori crumbs and roasted sesame seeds.

Transfer the bowl to the fridge and allow the salad to cool for at least 30 minutes.

Serve chilled and enjoy!

Nutrition:

Calories 409

Carbohydrates 7.1 g

Fats 38.25 g

Protein 7.6 g

## Artichoke White Bean Sandwich Spread

Preparation Time: 10 minutes

Servings: 2

**Ingredients:**

½ cup raw cashews, chopped

Water

1 clove garlic, cut into half

1 tablespoon lemon zest

1 teaspoon fresh rosemary, chopped

¼ teaspoon salt

¼ teaspoon pepper

6 tablespoons almond, soy or coconut milk

1 15.5-ounce can cannellini beans, rinsed and drained well

3 to 4 canned artichoke hearts, chopped

¼ cup hulled sunflower seeds

Green onions, chopped, for garnish

**Directions:**

Soak the raw cashews for 15 minutes in enough water to cover them.  Drain and dab with a paper towel to make them as dry as possible.

Transfer the cashews to a blender and add the garlic, lemon zest, rosemary, salt and pepper.  Pulse to break everything up and then add the milk, one tablespoon at a time, until the mixture is smooth and creamy.

Mash the beans in a bowl with a fork.  Add the artichoke hearts and sunflower seeds.  Toss to mix.

Pour the cashew mixture on top and season with more salt and pepper if desired.  Mix the ingredients well and spread on whole-wheat bread, crackers, or a wrap.

Nutrition:

Calories 110

Carbohydrates 14 g

Fats 4 g

Protein 6 g

**Buffalo Chickpea Wraps**
Preparation Time: 20 minutes

Cooking Time: 5 minutes

Servings: 4

**Ingredients:**

¼ cup plus 2 tablespoons hummus

2 tablespoons lemon juice

1½ tablespoons maple syrup

1 to 2 tablespoons hot water

1 head Romaine lettuce, chopped

1 15-ounce can chickpeas, drained, rinsed and patted dry

4 tablespoons hot sauce, divided

1 tablespoon olive or coconut oil

¼ teaspoon garlic powder

1 pinch sea salt

4 wheat tortillas

¼ cup cherry tomatoes, diced

¼ cup red onion, diced

¼ of a ripe avocado, thinly sliced

**Directions:**

Mix the hummus with the lemon juice and maple syrup in a large bowl.  Use a whisk and add the hot water, a little at a time until it is thick but spreadable.

Add the Romaine lettuce and toss to coat.  Set aside.

Pour the prepared chickpeas into another bowl.  Add three tablespoons of the hot sauce, the olive oil, garlic powder and salt; toss to coat.

Heat a metal skillet (cast iron works the best) over medium heat and add the chickpea mixture. Sauté for three to five minutes and mash gently with a spoon.

Once the chickpea mixture is slightly dried out, remove from the heat and add the rest of the hot sauce. Stir it in well and set aside.

Lay the tortillas on a clean, flat surface and spread a quarter cup of the buffalo chickpeas on top. Top with tomatoes, onion and avocado (optional) and wrap.

Nutrition:

Calories 254

Carbohydrates 39.4 g

Fats 6.7 g

Protein 9.1 g

## Coconut Veggie Wraps
Preparation Time: 5 minutes

Servings: 5

**Ingredients:**

1½ cups shredded carrots

1 red bell pepper, seeded, thinly sliced

2½ cups kale

1 ripe avocado, thinly sliced

1 cup fresh cilantro, chopped

5 coconut wraps

2/3 cups hummus

6½ cups green curry paste

**Directions:**

Slice, chop and shred all the vegetables.

Lay a coconut wrap on a clean flat surface and spread two tablespoons of the hummus and one tablespoon of the green curry paste on top of the end closest to you.

Place some carrots, bell pepper, kale and cilantro on the wrap and start rolling it up, starting from the edge closest to you.  Roll tightly and fold in the ends.

Place the wrap, seam down, on a plate to serve.

Nutrition:

Calories 236

Carbohydrates 23.6 g

Fats 14.3 g

Protein 5.5 g

**Cucumber Avocado Sandwich**
Preparation Time: 15 minutes

Servings: 2

**Ingredients:**

½ of a large cucumber, peeled, sliced

¼ teaspoon salt

4 slices whole-wheat bread

4 ounces goat cheese with or without herbs, at room temperature

2 Romaine lettuce leaves

1 large avocado, peeled, pitted, sliced

2 pinches lemon pepper

1 squeeze of lemon juice

½ cup alfalfa sprouts

**Directions:**

Peel and slice the cucumber thinly.  Lay the slices on a plate and sprinkle them with a quarter to a half teaspoon of salt.  Let this set for 10 minutes or until water appears on the plate.

Place the cucumber slices in a colander and rinse with cold water.  Let these drain, then place them on a dry plate and pat dry with a paper towel.

Spread all slices with goat cheese and place lettuce leaves on the two bottom pieces of bread.

Layer the cucumber slices and avocado atop the bread.

Sprinkle one pinch of lemon pepper over each sandwich and drizzle a little lemon juice over the top.

Top with the alfalfa sprouts and place another piece of bread, goat cheese down, on top.

Nutrition:

Calories 246

Carbohydrates 20 g

Fats 12 g

Protein 9 g

**Lentil Sandwich Spread**
Preparation Time: 15 minutes

Cooking Time: 20 minutes

Servings: 3

**Ingredients:**

1 tablespoon water or oil

1 small onion, chopped

2 cloves garlic, minced

1 cup dry lentils

2 cups vegetable stock

1 tablespoon apple cider vinegar

2 tablespoons tomato paste

3 sun-dried tomatoes

2 tablespoons maple

1 teaspoon dried oregano

½ teaspoon ground cumin

1 teaspoon coriander

1 teaspoon turmeric

½ lemon, juiced

1 tablespoon fresh parsley, chopped

**Directions:**

Warm a Dutch oven over medium heat and add the water or oil.

Immediately add the onions and sauté for two to three minutes or until softened.   Add more water if this starts to stick to the pan.

Add the garlic and sauté for one minute.

Add the lentils, vegetable stock and vinegar; bring to a boil. Turn down to a simmer and cook for 15 minutes or until the lentils are soft and the liquid is almost completely absorbed.

Ladle the lentils into a food processor and add the tomato paste, sun-dried tomatoes and syrup; process until smooth.

Add the oregano, cumin, coriander, turmeric and lemon; processes until thoroughly mixed.

Remove the spread to a bowl and apply it to bread, toast, a wrap, or pita. Sprinkle With toppings as desired.

Nutrition:

Calories 360

Carbohydrates 60.7 g

Fats 5.4 g

Protein 17.5 g

**Mediterranean Tortilla Pinwheels**
Preparation Time: 5 minutes

Cooking Time: 1 minute

Servings: 16

**Ingredients:**

½ cup water

4 tablespoons white vinegar

3 tablespoons lemon juice

3 tablespoons tahini paste

1 clove garlic, minced

Salt and pepper to taste

Canned artichokes, drained, thinly sliced

Cherry tomatoes, thinly sliced

Olives, thinly sliced

Lettuce or baby spinach

Tortillas

**Directions:**

In a bowl, combine the water, vinegar, lemon juice and
Tahini paste; whisk together until smooth.

Add the garlic, salt and pepper to taste; whisk to combine.  Set the bowl aside.

Lay a tortilla on a flat surface and spread with one tablespoon of the sauce.

Lay some lettuce or spinach slices on top, then scatter some artichoke, tomato and olive slices on top.

Tightly roll the tortilla and fold in the sides.  Cut the ends off and then slice into four or five pinwheels.

Nutrition:

Calories 322

Carbohydrates 5 g

Fats 4 g

Protein 30 g

**Rice and Bean Burritos**
Preparation Time: 10 minutes

Cooking Time: 15 minutes

Servings: 8

**Ingredients:**

2 16-ounce cans fat-free refried beans

6 tortillas

2 cups cooked rice

½ cup salsa

1 tablespoon olive oil

1 bunch green onions, chopped

2 bell peppers, finely chopped

Guacamole

**Directions:**

Preheat the oven to 375°F.

Dump the refried beans into a saucepan and place over medium heat to warm.

Heat the tortillas and lay them out on a flat surface.

Spoon the beans in a long mound that runs across the tortilla, just a little off from center.

Spoon some rice and salsa over the beans; add the green pepper and onions to taste, along with any other finely chopped vegetables you like.

Fold over the shortest edge of the plain tortilla and roll it up, folding in the sides as you go.

Place each burrito, seam side down, on a nonstick-sprayed baking sheet.

Brush with olive oil and bake for 15 minutes.

Serve with guacamole.

Nutrition:

Calories 290

Carbohydrates 49 g

Fats 6 g

Protein 9 g

# Dinner

## Summer Harvest Pizza

Preparation Time: 20 minutes

Cooking Time: 15 minutes

Servings: 2

**Ingredients:**

1 Lavash flatbread, whole grain

4 Tbsp Feta spread, store-bought

½ cup cheddar cheese, shredded

½ cup corn kernels, cooked

½ cup beans, cooked

½ cup fire-roasted red peppers, chopped

**Directions:**

Preheat oven to 350ºF.

Cut Lavash into two halves. Bake crusts on a pan in the oven for 5 minutes.

Spread feta spread on both crusts. Top with remaining ingredients.

Bake for another 10 minutes.

Nutrition:

Calories 230

Carbohydrates 23 g

Fats 15 g

Protein 11 g

**Whole Wheat Pizza with Summer Produce**
Preparation Time: 15 minutes

Cooking Time: 15 minutes

Servings: 2

**Ingredients:**

1 pound whole wheat pizza dough

4 ounces goat cheese

2/3 cup blueberries

2 ears corn, husked

2 yellow squash, sliced

2 Tbsp olive oil

**Directions:**

Preheat the oven to 450°F.

Roll the dough out to make a pizza crust.

Crumble the cheese on the crust. Spread remaining ingredients, then drizzle with olive oil.

Bake for about 15 minutes. Serve.

Nutrition:

Calories 470

Carbohydrates 66 g

Fats 18 g

Protein 17 g

**Spicy Chickpeas**
Preparation Time: 15 minutes

Cooking Time: 20 minutes

Servings: 8

**Ingredients:**

1 Tbsp extra-virgin olive oil

1 yellow onion, diced

1 tsp curry

¼ tsp allspice

1 can diced tomatoes

2 cans chickpeas, rinsed, drained

Salt, cayenne pepper, to taste

**Directions:**

Simmer onions in 1 Tbsp oil for 4 minutes.

Add allspice and pepper, cook for 2 minutes.

Stir in tomatoes, and cook for another 2 minutes.

Add chickpeas, and simmer for 10 minutes.

Season with salt, and serve.

Nutrition:

Calories 146

Carbohydrates 25 g

Fats 3 g

Protein 5 g

**Farro with Pistachios & Herbs**
Preparation Time: 20 minutes

Cooking Time: 45 minutes

Servings: 10

**Ingredients:**

2 cups farro

4 cups water

1 tsp kosher salt, divided

2½ Tbsp extra-virgin olive oil

1 onion, chopped

2 cloves garlic, minced

½ tsp ground pepper, divided

½ cup parsley, chopped

4 oz salted shelled pistachios, toasted, chopped

**Directions:**

Combine farro, water, and ¾ tsp salt, simmer for 40 minutes.

Cook onion and garlic in 2 Tbsp oil for 5 minutes.

Combine ½ tsp oil, ¼ tsp pepper, parsley, pistachios, and toss well.

Combine all. Season with salt and pepper.

Nutrition:

Calories 220

Carbohydrates 30 g

Fats 9 g

Protein 8 g

## Millet and Teff with Squash & Onions

Preparation Time: 10 minutes

Cooking Time: 20 minutes

Servings: 6

### Ingredients:

1 cup millet

½ cup teff grain

4½ cups of water

1 onion, sliced

1 butternut squash, chopped

Sea salt, to taste

### Directions:

Rinse millet, and put in a large pot.

Add remaining ingredients. Mix well.

Simmer 20 minutes until all the water is absorbed.

Serve hot.

Nutrition:

Calories 200

Carbohydrates 40 g

Fats 2 g

Protein 6 g

**Brown Rice Tabbouleh**
Preparation Time: 20 minutes

Cooking Time: 0 minutes

Servings: 6

**Ingredients:**

3 cups brown rice, cooked

¾ cup cucumber, chopped

¾ cup tomato, chopped

¼ cup mint leaves, chopped

¼ cup green onions, sliced

¼ cup olive oil

¼ cup lemon juice

Salt, pepper, to taste

**Directions:**

Combine all ingredients in a large bowl.

Toss well and chill for 20 min.

Nutrition:

Calories 201

Carbohydrates 25 g

Fats 10 g

Protein 3 g

**Healthy Hoppin' John**
Preparation Time: 15 minutes

Cooking Time: 1 hour

Servings: 4

**Ingredients:**

1 Tbsp extra-virgin olive oil

1 onion, diced

2 garlic cloves, minced

1 cup of dried black-eyed peas

1 cup brown rice, uncooked

4 cups water

Salt, pepper, to taste

**Directions:**

Cook the onions and garlic in oil for 3 minutes.

Combine the peas, salt, brown rice, and 4 cups of water and bring to a boil.

Add pepper. Simmer for 45 minutes.

Serve hot.

Nutrition:

Calories 248

Carbohydrates 47 g

Fats 5 g

Protein 6 g

**Beans & Greens Bowl**
Preparation Time: 2 minutes

Cooking Time: 2 minutes

Servings: 1

**Ingredients:**

1½ cups curly kale, washed, chopped

½ cup black beans, cooked

½ avocado

2 Tbsp feta cheese, crumbled

**Directions:**

Mix the kale and black beans in a microwavable bowl and heat for about 1 ½ minute.

Add the avocado and stir well. Top with feta.

Nutrition:

Calories 340

Carbohydrates 32 g

Fats 19 g

Protein 13 g

**Black Beans & Brown Rice**
Preparation Time: 2 minutes

Cooking Time: 45 minutes

Servings: 4

**Ingredients:**

4 cups water

2 cups brown rice, uncooked

1 can no-salt black beans

3 cloves garlic, minced

**Directions:**

Bring the water and rice to boil, simmer for 40 minutes.

In a pan, cook the black beans with their liquid and the garlic for 5 minutes.

Toss the rice and beans together, and serve.

Nutrition:

Calories 220

Carbohydrates 45 g

Fats 1.5 g

Protein 7 g

**Yucatan Bean & Pumpkin Seed Appetizer**
Preparation Time: 10 minutes

Cooking Time: 3 minutes

Servings: 8

**Ingredients:**

¼ cup pumpkin seeds

1 can white beans

1 tomato, chopped

1/3 cup onion, chopped

1/3 cup cilantro, chopped

4 Tbsp lime juice

Salt, pepper, to taste

**Directions:**

Toast the pumpkin seeds for 3 minutes to lightly brown. Let cool, and then chop in a food processor.

Mix in the remaining ingredients. Season with salt and pepper, and serve.

Nutrition:

Calories 12 g

Fats 2 g

Carbohydrates 12 g

Protein 5 g

**Butter Bean Hummus**
Preparation Time: 5 minutes

Cooking Time: 0 minutes

Servings: 4

**Ingredients:**

1 can butter beans, drained, rinsed

2 garlic cloves, minced

½ lemon, juiced

1 Tbsp olive oil

4 sprigs of parsley, minced

Sea salt, to taste

**Directions:**

Blend all ingredients in a food processor into a creamy mixture.

Serve as a dip for bread, crackers, or any types of vegetables.

Nutrition:

Calories 150

Carbohydrates 23 g

Fats 4 g

Protein 8 g

**Greek-style Gigante Beans**
Preparation Time: 8 hours 5 minutes

Cooking Time: 10 hours

Servings: 10

**Ingredients:**

12 ounces gigante beans

1 can tomatoes with juice, chopped

2 stalks celery, diced

1 onion, diced

4 garlic cloves, minced

Salt, to taste

**Directions:**

Soak beans in water for 8 hours.

Combine drained beans with the remaining ingredients. Stir, and pour water to cover.

Cook for 10 hours on low. Season with salt, and serve.

Nutrition:

Calories 63

Carbohydrates 13 g

Fats 2 g

Protein 4 g

**Brown Rice & Red Beans & Coconut Milk**
Preparation Time: 10 minutes

Cooking Time: 1 hour

Servings: 6

**Ingredients:**

2 cups brown rice, uncooked

4 cups water

1 Tbsp olive oil

1 onion, diced

3 cloves garlic, minced

2 cans red beans

1 can coconut milk

**Directions:**

Bring brown rice in water to a boil, then simmer for 30 minutes.

Sauté onion in olive oil. Add garlic and cook until golden.

Mix the onions and garlic, beans, and coconut milk into the rice. Simmer for 15 minutes.

Serve hot.

Nutrition:

Calories 280

Carbohydrates 49 g

Fats 3 g

Protein 8 g

**Black-Eyed Peas with Herns**
Preparation Time: 10 minutes

Cooking Time: 1 hour

Servings: 8

**Ingredients:**

2 cans no-sodium black-eyed beans

½ cup extra-virgin olive oil

1 cup parsley, chopped

4 green onions, sliced

2 carrots, grated

2 Tbsp tomato paste

2 cups water

Salt, pepper, to taste

**Directions:**

Drain the beans, reserve the liquid.

Sauté beans, parsley, onions, and carrots in oil for 3 minutes.

Add remaining ingredients, 2 cups reserved beans liquid, and water.

Cook for 30 minutes.

Season with salt, pepper and serve.

Nutrition:

Calories 230

Carbohydrates 23 g

Fats 15 g

Protein 11 g

# Snacks for Morning and Afternoon

## Nori Snack Rolls

Preparation Time: 5 Minutes

Cooking Time: 10 Minutes

Servings: 4 Rolls

## Ingredients

2 tablespoons almond, cashew, peanut, or other nut butter

2 tablespoons tamari, or soy sauce

4 standard nori sheets

1 mushroom, sliced

1 tablespoon pickled ginger

½ cup grated carrots

## Directions

Preheat the oven to 350°F.

Mix together the nut butter and tamari until smooth and very thick. Lay out a nori sheet, rough side up, the long way.

Spread a thin line of the tamari mixture on the far end of the nori sheet, from side to side. Lay the mushroom slices, ginger, and carrots in a line at the other end (the end closest to you).

Fold the vegetables inside the nori, rolling toward the tahini mixture, which will seal the roll. Repeat to make 4 rolls.

Put on a baking sheet and bake for 8 to 10 minutes, or until the rolls are slightly browned and crispy at the ends. Let the rolls cool for a few minutes, then slice each roll into 3 smaller pieces.

Per Serving (1 roll) Calories: 79; Total fat: 5g; Carbs: 6g; Fiber: 2g; Protein: 4g

## Kale Chips

Preparation Time: 5 Minutes

Cooking Time: 25 Minutes

Servings: 2

## Ingredients

1 large bunch kale

1 tablespoon extra-virgin olive oil

½ teaspoon chipotle powder

½ teaspoon smoked paprika

¼ teaspoon salt

## Directions

Preheat the oven to 275ºF.

Line a large baking sheet with parchment paper. In a large bowl, stem the kale and tear it into bite-size pieces. Add the olive oil, chipotle powder, smoked paprika, and salt.

Toss the kale with tongs or your hands, coating each piece well.

Spread the kale over the parchment paper in a single layer.

Bake for 25 minutes, turning halfway through, until crisp.

Cool for 10 to 15 minutes before dividing and storing in 2 airtight containers.

Nutrition: Calories: 144; Fat: 7g; Protein: 5g; Carbohydrates: 18g; Fiber: 3g; Sugar: 0g; Sodium: 363mg

**Savory Roasted Chickpeas**
Preparation Time: 5 Minutes

Cooking Time: 25 Minutes

Servings: 1 Cup

**Ingredients**

1 (14-ounce) can chickpeas, rinsed and drained, or 1½ cups cooked

2 tablespoons tamari, or soy sauce

1 tablespoon nutritional yeast

1 teaspoon smoked paprika, or regular paprika

1 teaspoon onion powder

½ teaspoon garlic powder

**Directions**

Preheat the oven to 400°F.

Toss the chickpeas with all the other ingredients, and spread them out on a baking sheet. Bake for 20 to 25 minutes, tossing halfway through.

Bake these at a lower temperature, until fully dried and crispy, if you want to keep them longer.

You can easily double the batch, and if you dry them out they will keep about a week in an airtight container.

Per Serving (¼ cup) Calories: 121; Total fat: 2g; Carbs: 20g; Fiber: 6g; Protein: 8g

**Savory Seed Crackers**
Preparation Time: 5 Minutes

Cooking Time: 50 Minutes

Servings: 20 Crackers

**Ingredients**

¾ cup pumpkin seeds (pepitas)

½ cup sunflower seeds

½ cup sesame seeds

¼ cup chia seeds

1 teaspoon minced garlic (about 1 clove)

1 teaspoon tamari or soy sauce

1 teaspoon vegan Worcestershire sauce

½ teaspoon ground cayenne pepper

½ teaspoon dried oregano

½ cup water

## Directions

Preheat the oven to 325ºF.

Line a rimmed baking sheet with parchment paper.

In a large bowl, combine the pumpkin seeds, sunflower seeds, sesame seeds, chia seeds, garlic, tamari, Worcestershire sauce, cayenne, oregano, and water.

Transfer to the prepared baking sheet, spreading out to all sides.

Bake for 25 minutes. Remove the pan from the oven, and flip the seed "dough" over so the wet side is up. Bake for another 20 to 25 minutes, until the sides are browned.

Cool completely before breaking up into 20 pieces. Divide evenly among 4 glass jars and close tightly with lids.

Per Serving (5 crackers): Calories: 339; Fat: 29g; Protein: 14g; Carbohydrates: 17g; Fiber: 8g; Sugar: 1g; Sodium: 96mg

## Lemon Coconut Cilantro Rolls
Preparation Time: 30 Minutes • Chill Time: 30 Minutes

Servings: 16 Pieces

## Ingredients

½ cup fresh cilantro, chopped

1 cup sprouts (clover, alfalfa)

1 garlic clove, pressed

2 tablespoons ground Brazil nuts or almonds

2 tablespoons flaked coconut

1 tablespoon coconut oil

Pinch cayenne pepper

Pinch sea salt

Pinch freshly ground black pepper

Zest and juice of 1 lemon

2 tablespoons ground flaxseed

1 to 2 tablespoons water

2 whole-wheat wraps, or corn wraps

**Directions**

Put everything but the wraps in a food processor and pulse to combine. Or combine the ingredients in a large bowl. Add the water, if needed, to help the mix come together.

Spread the mixture out over each wrap, roll it up, and place it in the fridge for 30 minutes to set.

Remove the rolls from the fridge and slice each into 8 pieces to serve as appetizers or sides with a soup or stew.

Get the best flavor by buying whole raw Brazil nuts or almonds, toasting them lightly in a dry skillet or toaster oven, and then grinding them in a coffee grinder.

Per Serving (1 piece) Calories: 66; Total fat: 4g; Carbs: 6g; Fiber: 1g; Protein: 2g

**Tamari Almonds**
Preparation Time: 5 Minutes

Cooking Time: 15 Minutes

Servings: 8

**Ingredients**

1 pound raw almonds

3 tablespoons tamari or soy sauce

2 tablespoons extra-virgin olive oil

1 tablespoon nutritional yeast

1 to 2 teaspoons chili powder, to taste

**Directions**

Preheat the oven to 400ºF.

Line a baking sheet with parchment paper.

In a medium bowl, combine the almonds, tamari, and olive oil until well coated.

Spread the almonds on the prepared baking sheet and roast for 10 to 15 minutes, until browned.

Cool for 10 minutes, then season with the nutritional yeast and chili powder.

Transfer to a glass jar and close tightly with a lid.

Nutrition: Calories: 364; Fat: 32g; Protein: 13g; Carbohydrates: 13g; Fiber: 7g; Sugar: 3g; Sodium: 381mg

**Tempeh Taco Bites**
PREPARATION TIME: 5 MINUTES

Cooking Time: 45 MINUTES

Servings: 3 Dozen

**Ingredients**

8 ounces tempeh

3 tablespoons soy sauce

2 teaspoons ground cumin

1 teaspoon chili powder

1 teaspoon dried oregano

1 tablespoon olive oil

1/2 cup finely minced onion

2 garlic cloves, minced

Salt and freshly ground black pepper

2 tablespoons tomato paste

1 chipotle chile in adobo, finely minced

1/4 cup hot water or vegetable broth, homemade or store-bought, plus more if needed

36 phyllo pastry cups, thawed

1/2 cup basic guacamole, homemade or store-bought

18 ripe cherry tomatoes, halved

**Directions**

In a medium saucepan of simmering water, cook the tempeh for 30 minutes. Drain well, then finely mince and place it in a bowl. Add the soy sauce, cumin, chili powder, and oregano. Mix well and set aside.

In a medium skillet, heat the oil over medium heat. Add the onion, cover, and cook for 5 minutes. Stir in the garlic, then add the tempeh mixture and cook, stirring, for 2 to 3 minutes. Season with salt and pepper to taste. Set aside.

In a small bowl, combine the tomato paste, chipotle, and the hot water or broth. Return tempeh mixture to heat and in stir tomato-chile mixture and cook for 10 to 15 minutes, stirring occasionally, until the liquid is absorbed. The mixture should be fairly dry, but if it begins to stick to the pan, add a little hotter water, 1 tablespoon at a time. Taste, adjusting seasonings if necessary. Remove from the heat.

To assemble, fill the phyllo cups to the top with the tempeh filling, using about 2 teaspoons of filling in each. Top with a dollop of guacamole and a cherry tomato half and serve.

## Mushroom Croustades

Preparation Time: 10 Minutes

Cooking Time: 10 Minutes

Servings: 12 Croustades

### Ingredients

12 thin slices whole-grain bread

1 tablespoon olive oil, plus more for brushing bread

2 medium shallots, chopped

2 garlic cloves, minced

12 ounces white mushrooms, chopped

1/4 cup chopped fresh parsley

1 teaspoon dried thyme

1 tablespoon soy sauce

**Directions**

Preheat the oven to 400°F. Using a 3-inch round pastry cutter or a drinking glass, cut a circle from each bread slice. Brush the bread circles with oil and press them firmly but gently into a mini-muffin tin. Bake until the bread is toasted, about 10 minutes.

Meanwhile, in a large skillet, heat the 1 tablespoon oil over medium heat. Add the shallots, garlic, and mushrooms and sauté for 5 minutes to soften the vegetables. Stir in the parsley, thyme, and soy sauce and cook until the liquid is absorbed, about 5 minutes longer. Spoon the mushroom mixture into the croustade cups and return to the oven for 3 to 5 minutes to heat through. Serve warm.

**Stuffed Cherry Tomatoes**
Preparation Time: 15 Minutes

Cooking Time: 0 Minutes

Servings: 6

**Ingredients**

2 pints cherry tomatoes, tops removed and centers scooped out

2 avocados, mashed

juice of 1 lemon

½ red bell pepper, minced

4 green onions (white and green parts), finely minced

1 tablespoon minced fresh tarragon

pinch of sea salt

**Directions**

Place the cherry tomatoes open-side up on a platter.

In a small bowl, combine the avocado, lemon juice, bell pepper, scallions, tarragon, and salt.

Stir until well combined. Scoop into the cherry tomatoes and serve immediately.

**Spicy Black Bean Dip**
Preparation Time: 10 Minutes

Cooking Time: 0 Minutes

Servings: 2 Cups

**Ingredients**

1 (14-ounce) can black beans, drained and rinsed, or 1½ cups cooked

Zest and juice of 1 lime

1 tablespoon tamari, or soy sauce

¼ cup water

¼ cup fresh cilantro, chopped

1 teaspoon ground cumin

Pinch cayenne pepper

**Directions**

Put the beans in a food processor (best choice) or blender, along with the lime zest and juice, tamari, and about ¼ cup of water.

Blend until smooth, then blend in the cilantro, cumin, and cayenne.

If you don't have a blender or prefer a different consistency, simply transfer it to a bowl once the beans have been puréed and stir in the spices, instead of forcing the blender.

Per Serving (1 cup) Calories: 190; Total fat: 1g; Carbs: 35g; Fiber: 12g; Protein: 13g

**French Onion Pastry Puffs**
Preparation Time: 10 Minutes

Cooking Time: 35 Minutes - Makes 24 Puffs

**Ingredients**

2 tablespoons olive oil

2 medium onions, thinly sliced

1 garlic clove, minced

1 teaspoon chopped fresh rosemary

Salt and freshly ground black pepper

1 tablespoon capers

1 sheet frozen vegan puff pastry, thawed

18 pitted black olives, quartered

**Directions**

In a medium skillet, heat the oil over medium heat. Add the onions and garlic, season with rosemary and salt and pepper to taste. Cover and cook until very soft, stirring occasionally, about 20 minutes. Stir in the capers and set aside.

Preheat the oven to 400°F. Roll out the puff pastry and cut into 2- to 3-inch circles using a lightly floured pastry cutter or drinking glass. You should get about 2 dozen circles.

Arrange the pastry circles on baking sheets and top each with a heaping teaspoon of onion mixture, patting down to smooth the top.

Top with 3 olive quarters, arranged decoratively—either like flower petals emanating from the center or parallel to each other like 3 bars.

Bake until pastry is puffed and golden brown, about 15 minutes. Serve hot.

**Cheezy Cashew–Roasted Red Pepper Toasts**
Preparation Time: 15 Minutes

Cooking Time: 0 Minutes

Servings: 16 To 24 Toasts

## Ingredients

2 jarred roasted red peppers

1 cup unsalted cashews

1/4 cup water

1 tablespoon soy sauce

2 tablespoons chopped green onions

1/4 cup nutritional yeast

2 tablespoons balsamic vinegar

2 tablespoons olive oil

## Directions

Use canapé or cookie cutters to cut the bread into desired shapes about 2 inches wide. If you don't have a cutter, use a knife to cut the bread into squares, triangles, or rectangles. You should get 2 to 4 pieces out of each slice of bread. Toast the bread and set aside to cool.

Coarsely chop 1 red pepper and set aside. Cut the remaining pepper into thin strips or decorative shapes and set aside for garnish.

In a blender or food processor, grind the cashews to a fine powder. Add the water and soy sauce and process until smooth. Add the chopped red pepper and puree. Add the green onions, nutritional yeast, vinegar, and oil and process until smooth and well blended.

Spread a spoonful of the pepper mixture onto each of the toasted bread pieces and top decoratively with the reserved pepper strips. Arrange on a platter or tray and serve.

## Baked Potato Chips

Preparation Time: 10 Minutes

Cooking Time: 30 Minutes

Servings: 4

**Ingredients**

1 large Russet potato

1 teaspoon paprika

½ teaspoon garlic salt

¼ teaspoon vegan sugar

¼ teaspoon onion powder

¼ teaspoon chipotle powder or chili powder

⅛ teaspoon salt

⅛ teaspoon ground mustard

⅛ teaspoon ground cayenne pepper

1 teaspoon canola oil

⅛ teaspoon liquid smoke

**Directions**

Wash and peel the potato. Cut into thin, 1/10-inch slices (a mandoline slicer or the slicer blade in a food processor is helpful for consistently sized slices).

Fill a large bowl with enough very cold water to cover the potato. Transfer the potato slices to the bowl and soak for 20 minutes.

Preheat the oven to 400ºF. Line a baking sheet with parchment paper.

In a small bowl, combine the paprika, garlic salt, sugar, onion powder, chipotle powder, salt, mustard, and cayenne.

Drain and rinse the potato slices and pat dry with a paper towel.

Transfer to a large bowl.

Add the canola oil, liquid smoke, and spice mixture to the bowl. Toss to coat.

Transfer the potatoes to the prepared baking sheet.

Bake for 15 minutes. Flip the chips over and bake for 15 minutes longer, until browned. Transfer the chips to 4 storage containers or large glass jars.

Let cool before closing the lids tightly.

Nutrition: Calories: 89; Fat: 1g; Protein: 2g; Carbohydrates: 18g; Fiber: 2g; Sugar: 1g; Sodium: 65mg

# *Chapter 7 Let's go shopping*

Now that we have a good understanding of the nutritional value of plant-based foods, let us go to the supermarket to stock the cupboards, fridge, and freezer with everything we need to get this new lifestyle started.

Every supermarket is laid out in a similar way, so this list will be designed to make it as easy as possible for you to get what you need and navigate the layout with ease. There will always be a fresh produce section which usually is the first area you come across but is sometimes the last.  It is always to one side of the supermarket.  The dairy fridges are usually close by to the produce, along with the vegetarian fridges.  The health foods aisle will be adjacent to the produce section along with the bulk bins.

The middle aisles of the supermarket are always reserved for convenience and junk foods, cereals, and packet meals.  The personal care and cleaning products follow the rice, pasta, canned foods, and baking supplies, then comes the freezer aisles and bakery.  Let's begin!

FRESH PRODUCE

Anything in this department is available to you as it is all fruits and vegetables.  Take your time getting to know each area from the berries to the citrus, root vegetables to the leafy greens.  It is recommended not to overwhelm yourself at first, so stick to what you know and every visit, pick up something you haven't tried before and given it a go.  You'll find new favorite foods and ones you don't like so much, but it's all part of the fun!

FRUIT

Citrus fruits: Lemons, oranges, limes, grapefruit, mandarins.

Stone fruits: Peaches, plums, nectarines, cherries, apricots

Melons: Watermelon, honeydew, cantaloupe

Berries: Strawberries, raspberries, blueberries, blackberries, gooseberries, kiwi

Tropical fruits: Banana, mango, pineapple, papaya, dragon fruit, lychee, coconut, passionfruit

Apples and pears: Granny Smith, Braeburn, golden delicious, red delicious, pink lady, gala, Fuji, McIntosh.

Dates and figs: you will find fresh in the produce aisle.

VEGETABLES

Roots: Potato, sweet potato, yam, carrot, beets, celeriac, radish, parsnip, ginger, turmeric, turnip.

Bulbs: Garlic, onion, shallots, green onion.

Stems: Celery, asparagus, rhubarb.

Marrows: Pumpkin, acorn squash, spaghetti squash, gem squash.

Cruciferous: Broccoli, cauliflower, Brussel sprouts, cabbage.

Leafy greens: Lettuce, spinach, collard greens, chard, arugula, kale, bok choy, watercress.

Peppers: Bell, chili, jalapeno, habanero, banana pepper.

Other: Mushrooms, cucumber, zucchini, eggplant, tomato, cherry tomato artichoke, avocado, beans, peas, corn, sprouts.

FRESH HERBS:

Leafy herbs: Basil, cilantro, parsley, mint.

Cooking herbs: Marjoram, oregano, sage, thyme, rosemary, anise, caraway, bay leaves, kaffir lime leaves.

Accompaniment herbs: Dill, chives, fennel, lavender.

DRIED FOODS

These foods are mainly fruits, herbs, and spices and also apply to the bulk bin sections, which are a great way to try new foods and flavors without paying much money or worrying that you'll be stuck with a huge amount of something you won't like.

Nuts: Almonds, brazil nuts, cashews, hazelnuts, macadamias, pecans, pistachios, pine nuts, walnuts.

Seeds: Chia seeds, flax seeds, flaxseed meal, hemp hearts, sesame seeds, sunflower seeds, pumpkin seeds, hemp hearts.

Dried Fruit: Apricots, dates, figs, mulberries, cranberries, raisins, blueberries, banana chips, mango, goji berries, shredded coconut, desiccated coconut.

Dried Herbs: Basil, celery seed, cloves, coriander seeds, dill, Italian herbs, oregano, parsley, rosemary, sage, thyme.

Dried Spices: Black pepper, cardamom, chili powder, chili flakes, cinnamon, cumin, curry powder, garlic powder, nutmeg, onion powder, paprika, turmeric.

Salt: Sea salt, pink Himalayan salt, black salt.

Dried legumes: Black beans, chickpeas, red kidney beans, white kidney beans, pinto beans, lentils, cannellini beans.

Other: Nutritional yeast, kelp flakes, dried seaweed, nori sheets, rice paper rounds.

CANNED FOODS

This aisle is a haven for a vegan with so many whole food options that can be kept in a pantry for emergencies, additions to meals and has a very long shelf life. Obviously fresh foods are better for you but rotating canned foods into your diet will help ensure you have enough options to keep you happy on this new lifestyle.

The following is a recommended list of handy and delicious items that work well in recipes.  If you have a favorite canned vegetable or fruit that is not on this list, please continue to enjoy it.

Vegetables:  Diced/chopped tomatoes, tomato puree, corn, pumpkin puree, beets.

Fruits:  Coconut milk, coconut cream, peaches, pears, pineapple, apples, jackfruit.

Legumes:  Black beans, lentils, red kidney beans, white kidney beans, pinto beans, chickpeas, cannellini beans, butter beans, bean salad, vegan refried beans (caution as a lot of refried beans contain pork lard)

JAR GOODS:

Often better than canned goods due to being stored in glass rather than tin.  There are many amazing food items in this area that should be kept and savored in your fridge or pantry.  They are often richer in flavor than their fresh counterparts and marinated in herbs, spices, and oils that complement meals very well.

Vegetables: Olives, sundried tomatoes, pickles, banana peppers, roasted red peppers, salsa, sauerkraut, capers, artichoke hearts.

Fruit: Applesauce, high-quality whole jams or spreads.

NUT AND SEED BUTTERS

You won't be sorry you found this aisle.  These butters are full of concentrated proteins, fibers, and vitamins and are essential to recipes at any meal of the day from smoothies to satays to desserts.

Nut Butters: Almond butter, cashew butter, hazelnut butter, peanut butter, peanut and coconut butter, macadamia butter, walnut butter.

Seed Butters: Pumpkin seed butter, sunflower seed butter, tahini.

GRAINS

Grains can be found in multiple areas of the grocery store.  The cheaper items can be found in the bulk section, the higher priced items will be found in the health food aisle and they can also be found in the baking aisle.  It is recommended that you take your time finding the brands and types that work for you, but if you are trying something for the first time, start in the bulk section.

Rice: White rice, brown rice, wild rice, basmati rice, jasmine rice, long grain rice, short grain rice, saffron rice.

Pasta: Linguine, spaghetti, penne, macaroni, lasagna, cannelloni, shell pasta. (most of these can be found in whole wheat varieties to up the nutrient factor and there are also very good gluten-free pasta brands now too)

Oats: Rolled oats, quick oats, steel-cut oats.

Grains: Amaranth, bulgur wheat, barley, couscous, quinoa, buckwheat, millet.

Other: Popcorn.

BAKING AND COOKING

There are many items in this aisle that are essential to creating dishes to help you recreate favorite meals from before this transition.  There are also a lot of processed and refined items that are damaging to your health.  Do your best to choose the whole-grain, raw and whole varieties as much as possible.

Flour:  All-purpose, almond, buckwheat, chickpea, coconut, whole wheat, rice flour.

Baking: Arrowroot powder, tapioca starch, potato starch, corn starch, baking powder, baking soda, agar-agar, cocoa powder, cacao powder.

Sugar: Raw sugar, brown sugar, coconut sugar, blackstrap molasses.

Sweeteners: Maple syrup, agave syrup, stevia.

Other: Vegan chocolate chips, vegan cooking chocolate, cacao nibs, vanilla extract.

SAUCES, OILS, AND CONDIMENTS

One of the most important aisles for cooking vegan meals.  There are many ethnic and cultural items that you may have never heard of before but are packed with flavor.  Be cautious of fish sauce or seafood ingredients in Asian sauces and flavorings.

Vinegars: Balsamic vinegar, red wine vinegar, white wine vinegar, rice wine vinegar, apple cider vinegar, malt vinegar.

Oils: Avocado oil, olive oil, coconut oil, sesame oil, peanut oil, sunflower oil, hemp oil, flax oil, walnut oil, canola oil, coconut cooking spray.

Condiments: Ketchup, Dijon mustard, yellow mustard, whole grain mustard, vegan mayonnaise, sriracha, hot sauce, sweet chili sauce.

Sauces: Soy sauce, coconut amino, tamari (gf).

Others: Miso Paste

FREEZER SECTION

A great place to find staple items that come in very handy when you've run out of fresh produce or want to keep something fresh that you use often.

Vegetables: Mixed, peas, carrots, corn, spinach, broccoli, cauliflower rice, avocado

Fruit: Mixed berries, blueberries, raspberries, strawberries, blackberries, smoothie mix, mango, banana, cranberries, cherries.

Meat Substitutes: Vegan mince, vegan burger patties, vegan chicken filets.

Other: Phyllo pastry, puff pastry (just check the ingredients for oil instead of butter)

CHILLED SECTION

Some supermarkets keep the vegan items next to the dairy items, whereas other supermarkets will keep the vegan fridges next to the fresh produce. Take your time getting acquainted with your own supermarket.

Milk: Almond milk, coconut milk, cashew milk, rice milk, oat milk, hemp milk, soymilk.

Cheese: Vegan sour cream, vegan cream cheese.

There are many great vegan kinds of cheese out there ranging from soy cheese to nut cheese. There is also a great variety of types from shredded, blocks, creams, and slices.

Yogurt: Coconut yogurt, almond yogurt, soy yogurt, cashew yogurt.

Butter: Vegan margarine (used as margarine and also for cooking and baking)

Meat substitutes: Veggie burgers, breakfast patties, vegan sausages, deli slices.

Other: Silky tofu, extra firm tofu, coconut water, orange juice.

BAKERY

Lots of goodies in this section that are not what you want in your cupboard or that contain dairy or eggs. If you stick to the edges of this section and avoid the cases, you should navigate yourself quite easily.

Bread: Sourdough loaf, rye bread, multigrain bread, unsliced bakery loaf, baguettes, bagels, English muffins. (some bread contains egg or milk so check the labels)

Wraps: Large tortilla, mini tortillas, corn tortillas.

OTHER:

Extras that are usually found in the health food aisle.

Vegan protein powder

Vegan protein bars

Spirulina

Greens powder

TIPS AND TRICKS AT THE GROCERY STORE:

The number one hardest thing about going vegan can be a sense of loss.  We are creatures of habit and we get used to having the things we like, so when these things are taken away and not replaced with something else, the sense of grief will derail our commitments and see us reaching for what we promised ourselves we would give up.

So, how do we avoid this from happening when going vegan?  You've already accomplished the first part which is educating ourselves on why we are giving up the meat, dairy and eggs and positive reasons for how doing so will improve our lives.

The second part is to make sure we don't feel like we've given anything up. The best way to do this is by taking a hard look at your previous diet. Write down what your favorite meals are, what you would take for lunch, what you would have for breakfast every day, and most importantly, what were your favorite treats. Once you have this written down, try to find reasons as to why you have chosen these foods and meals. Is it because they taste good? Or remind you of something? Do they make you feel a certain way when you're done? Full, or satisfied, energized or guilty? Once you've figured this part out, you might begin to understand your relationship with food a little better.

Now, we need to find vegan replacements for these meals and food items that will replicate these feelings, so you never feel like you're missing out.

For example:

You usually have a fried egg and white toast with butter for breakfast because it's quick to make and fills you up and is simple. You might really enjoy switching to avocado toast instead. The avocado will mimic the egg and butter in fat content, and a sprinkle of hemp or chia seeds on top will help to replace the protein from the egg. You could switch your white toast for a good quality whole wheat toast that will keep you fuller for longer but still takes the same amount of time to make.  A sprinkle of nutritional yeast will and sea salt with black pepper will keep it tasty and you happy.

You only eat tuna salad sandwiches for lunch with a packet of chips.  Switch the tuna salad for a chickpea salad that you can make ahead of time.  Make sure you have a delicious soft whole wheat bread or bun to satisfy the carb side of this equation.  Find a good quality root vegetable chip to tide you over while you slowly switch this to a nut and seed snack mix and maybe some sliced veggie sticks.

Your afternoon snack is always yogurt and chocolate biscuits.  There are fantastic coconut or almond yogurts out there now!  Try a few to find a good replacement that has a similar taste to your old favorite.  Maybe trade your chocolate biscuit for a trail mix that has some pretzels and vegan chocolate chips in there.

You adore chips and dip and can't imagine giving that up at night while you watch TV.  Okay!  Maybe keep the chips for now but sub the dip for homemade guacamole or hummus.  Slowly incorporate veggie sticks and delicious seed crackers into the mix as you slowly pull the chips out of your nighttime routine.

As you can see, there are so many ways to trick yourself into a new diet and lifestyle.  Please just be patient with yourself, love yourself for trying to be healthier, and keep reminding yourself of all the good that is about to come your way with this new way of being.

# *Conclusion*

A Plant-based meal is a very good substitute for the normal meals that we have. It has a number of advantages that have been discussed in this booklet, as well as its fair share of challenges and the best way that you can beat them to incorporate a happy and fulfilling eating style. With a plant-based meal plan, any individual is able to beat a number of chronic diseases that are brought forth with the type of eating lifestyle that we all hold. Life is intense, severe and unforgiving. This book has been tailor-made for beginners who would like to start on a plant-based meal plans as it emphasizes on the advantages and reasons as to why we should take plant-based meals and having listed the reasons as to why vegetables are better than meat. Vegetables are known to reduce the risks of some diseases, and hence even the medical technicians do encourage that even for non-vegetarians that they should add a little bit more vegetables in their diets more than the meat or animal products. This book has listed down the types of food to avoid once one has started off with a plant-based meal plan so as to make the most out of the plant products. For beginners, the book is well furnished with the knowledge of the basics of a plant-based meal plan and how to go about it and stick to it.

Understanding the benefits of a plant-based meal plan to our body is essential. This book is well equipped with the benefits that impact us positively in our bodies once we choose to start taking more of plant-based meals. Having listed a number of health benefits, it is a big challenge for one to stick to one meal plan and hence the challenges and temptations of seeing other people enjoy animal products and not getting tempted to have a taste of it. This is covered in this book as a cheat day; this is the only day that one is allowed to eat a non-plant meal just for a day. One would decide to eat meat and animal product that are not similar to the ones that are in the plant-based meal plan. A plant-based meal plan will assist in a number of things, including reducing weight as well as improving the general health of the skin. This book is equipped with a monthly meal plan that will assist a beginner to follow and introduce themselves into a plant-based meal plan as a lot of people find it as a challenge on how a what to prepare as meals once they switch to a plant meal based eating plan.

The focal point of this work is to encourage people to consume a lot of plant products by noting down the importance and challenges that people with this kind of diets go through and giving solutions on how to beat them and lead a healthy lifestyle that will encourage them to eat a lot of plant-based meals. The knowledge in this booklet will assist anyone to lead a healthy and disease-free life.